Praise for *In Search of You*

"Kasey takes us on her journey to finding joy through relatable (and captivating!) life stories coupled with thought-provoking self-reflection questions for readers. You'll finish this book finding your JOY and nurturing your inner child."
—Maureen Werrbach, LCPC, owner of Urban Wellness and The Group Practice Exchange

"Kasey Compton beautifully intertwines self-discovery with healing from life's traumas. This book is an invaluable guide for finding light regardless of your life's path so far."
—Melissa Dlugolecki, grief expert

"In *In Search of You*, Kasey Compton eloquently echoes what I've observed throughout my career: the essential connection between self-love and genuine contentment. As a leading expert in stored emotions and trauma in the body and providing a clear path forward for health and wholeness, I wholeheartedly endorse this transformative book."
—Aimie Apigian, MD, founder of Biology of Trauma® Model

In Search of You

How to Find Joy When Doing More Isn't Doing It Anymore

KASEY COMPTON

BENBELLA

BenBella Books, Inc.
Dallas, TX

BenBella Books, Inc.
10440 N. Central Expressway
Suite 800
Dallas, TX 75231
benbellabooks.com
Send feedback to feedback@benbellabooks.com

BenBella is a federally registered trademark.

Printed in the United States of America
10 9 8 7 6 5 4 3 2 1

Library of Congress Control Number: 2023041948
ISBN 9781637744444 (trade paperback)
ISBN 9781637744451 (electronic)

Editing by Gregory Newton Brown
Copyediting by Elizabeth Degenhard
Proofreading by Marissa Wold Uhrina and Rebecca Maines
Text design and composition by PerfecType
Cover design by Brigid Pearson
Printed by Lake Book Manufacturing

Special discounts for bulk sales are available. Please contact bulkorders@benbellabooks.com.

This book is for my girls. *All* of them.

Contents

PART FIVE | *Change*

CONCLUSION | *Choosing Joy*

Letter to You, Reader

Dear Reader,

This book was written, for the most part, in real time—part journal entry, part therapy assignment, part excavated memories. Some of the stories still feel raw. I never expected anyone to read my thoughts or revelations at first. In fact, I wanted to keep them locked away in a drawer for the rest of my life. It wasn't until I realized the change that was happening inside of me and the profound impact that my newfound vulnerability had, not just on me but on those I love, that I knew I needed to share them with others.

Starting now. Starting with you.

I always wished for a close friend, sister, or mentor who knew what I was going through, someone who could offer me wisdom and strength, and advise me on my next steps. It was always a missing piece in my life. I've never had a bestie with whom I could sit on the back porch drinking a cold glass of sweet tea, and I always wanted that. Someone who gets me—someone who understands and loves me—no matter what.

I can't help but believe that if I had had someone like that years ago, when I was going through so much internal turmoil, the path I took toward joy would have been much different.

But, nevertheless, in my long journey toward finding fulfillment, I found it and so much more. This book details that journey, mainly how I rediscovered myself and filled the emptiness with happiness, invited more vitality into my life, and began to see myself as a blessing to others and, more importantly, to myself.

I do want to clarify one thing so there's no confusion before you read any further.

This book, this process, this journey is not just about past hardships and trauma. It's not about dredging up your childhood and adulthood hurts so you can fix the pain, but that might happen. Please know, in our search together, we will go to heavier places, but at the end of the day, it's about joy.

Your joy.

Finding it, choosing it, understanding it, and hanging on to it.

We'll do that by looking back over your life and remembering the people and Big Things that made an impact on you. Then we'll move into the Little Things that show up in patterns—in repeated mistakes. We'll go deeper into *all* those things so you can develop a fuller sense of awareness and become more attuned to them. Finally, we'll seek to Understand what it all means. Because then, and only then, true change can occur—only when you come toe to toe with what you've needed to face all along can you see what's missing from your life.

I hope the wisdom you pick up from my personal stories helps you create the space within your own heart to feel whole. So, friend, pour yourself a glass of something sweet and come get lost in the pages, the words, and the memories with me. Remember, this is the first step in a journey to discover not only who you truly are, but who you were always meant to be.

Your New Back Porch Bestie,
Kasey

P.S. You may be feeling a lot of uncertainty as you embark on this quest, but I'd like to support you and follow up throughout your journey. If you're serious about exploring yourself and finding inner joy, I'd like to invite you to email me and let me know. I've set up a new email account solely to receive correspondence from readers like you: seeker@kaseycompton.com.

I read and respond to all my emails, so even if it takes me a few days to reply, know that I'm here cheering you on.

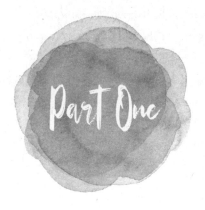

The Turning Point

• When you are willing to feel, you can heal. •

"Be brave enough to heal yourself
even when it hurts.
Most of your strength lies in your scars."
~Bianca Sparacino, author of *Seeds Planted in Concrete* and *The Strength in Our Scars*

Time is hard. It can be our greatest love *or* worst enemy. It can be on our side *or* work against us. Some might call a certain point in time a watershed moment or a turning point, but it's often a secret revelation, one that happens slowly, sometimes without you even knowing. It can be a choice between two pains—one you know is right, one you know will hurt. Make that choice, reader, regardless of what it is, because standing still only hurts worse in the end.

The Party—July 19, 2021

The sounds of party guests spill from my great room, through the confines of my bedroom, and into the deepest end of my closet, where I stand paralyzed by indecision. My Granny Sylvia used to tell me I was as jumpy as a long-tailed cat in a room full of rocking chairs, and that's certainly how I feel right now. Each time the front door opens and closes, I reach out and steady myself against the opposite wall.

I bought six dresses for this occasion, and I try each one of them on twice. *Nope, this one is too low-cut. Nuh uh, this one is too short. Shit, I must have lost weight since I bought this.* The sheer black one with lace and a rose-colored slip is as classy as I can muster. *Thank God I ordered it.* Nothing fits me anymore. Nothing feels right on my figure. Nothing matches my mood. I feel more like Elly May Clampett on an episode of *The Beverly Hillbillies*, tryin' to fit into something, to be someone, someplace I don't belong.

I stare at the outline of a body in the full-length mirror and barely recognize it. You'd think thirty pounds lighter would be a good thing, but for me, it's not. I'm tired but I still manage to crawl into the Spanx jumpsuit I never needed until I had my third baby, then I drop the dress down over my disheveled hair. I pluck the black pumps from the shoe rack and tell myself I can do this. I pray that for my guests, at least, I look better than I feel.

I walk into the bathroom to take a brush to my hair. Jessi, an employee of one of my businesses, walks in unexpectedly. It's so like her to see a closed door and walk through it with no thought to what's going on behind it. "Damn, girl," she says with a giggle.

I'm surprised to see her standing there. She looks surprised right back. I realize no one has seen me dressed up in months. I've barely left the house.

I quickly hide my discomfort with a question. "Do you think I need to curl my hair or leave it straight?" I never wear it straight, but the thought of running a curling iron through it feels like too much work.

She shakes her head and tells me it looks good the way it is, so I leave it. That's one less thing I must do. I'm already late. I spray a single pump of Love Spell body mist from the second drawer below the sink. I inhale deeply until I have nowhere else to put the air. I'm nervous about facing my guests, but I know I must. After all, they're here to celebrate my big accomplishment. Today I launch my first book.

This is the moment I have been waiting for—working for. The last big shiny object that I have spent my life chasing—becoming an author is what I have dreamed of since I was nine years old and operated a library from my mom's second-floor apartment. Housing all the books was a pink bookshelf handmade by my Poppy—a gift for learning to read.

And today, *I am* an author. At thirty-seven years old, my dream has come true.

I walk through the pocket door robotically, leaving the bathroom and moving past my bed covered with discarded clothes and slews of scattered suitcases. I hear the buzz of voices and listen to footsteps as they move back and forth from my kitchen to the porch, the one that spans the length of my entire house. I see their outlines from the window of my bedroom as I leave the room.

I slip into the living room and touch the wall where the collage of pictures from my parents' wedding day, some fifty-odd years ago, hangs. I see friends enjoying the enormous charcuterie board, a couple of colleagues from the office chit-chatting, and my oldest daughter, Maime, stuffing a green olive into her mouth. I smell the goat cheese and blueberry jam, of all things. The Kentucky bourbon is strong; the wind that blows in from the outside brings a trace of oak straight into my nose and leaves me yearning for one of my favorite drinks, an old fashioned. My senses are all alive and awake, even if my heart feels like it's barely beating.

The bartender standing to the side recognizes my desire.

"I make a delicious chocolate old fashioned with orange peel, and my margaritas are to die for," he says.

"I'll have one of each."

With drinks in hand, I think about how I wish I'd had one of these while getting ready. I continue to scan the room. My eyes are drawn to a long table stacked with decorative boxes and a mound of my books on display. *My* books. It's the perfect centerpiece for the occasion. I see my author headshot that I initially resisted sneering at me from the back, and I can't help but giggle a little.

I take it all in. I think about the people and things that have influenced me, and when I see the vintage German shepherd bookends sitting atop the cabinets I had made after I bought the house, I stop to breathe. Custom-made watercolor artwork that showcased my dream house on the hill, the one that I'm standing in at this very moment, calls the middle shelf its home. My children's piercing blue eyes stare at me from the printed canvases spread across the walls. They're so beautiful. My house is beautiful.

I think back on the time when I was nearly homeless and was forced to file bankruptcy because of a broken-down car I could no longer afford. I think about living in that small house on Richardson Drive that was infested with mold while working a second job as a restaurant server just to pay for Maime's preschool. I think about how far I have come, how I promised myself I would create a better life than the one I had growing up, and how, for the most part, I have. In the last twelve years I have overcome nearly every struggle one could have, from major health scares to financial destitution, and here I am living, breathing proof that dreams can come true.

My mentors couldn't make it to the party live, so they Zoomed in to congratulate me in front of my guests, and I'm relieved. I don't know if I could have managed to hide my feelings from them if they were here in person. They would know something is off—they would see my discomfort. Now, they are here virtually, waiting for me to appear.

I force a smile into my laptop camera, which is hooked up to the big screen television, and they applaud me heartily. I know what that means. I've done it. The degree. The career. The family. The businesses. The money. The vacation home.

The savings account. The college fund. I've done *everything* I set out to do, and they congratulate me for that.

Behind me, the girls from work surround the bartender and laugh. I hear the clink of ice as they raise their glasses in celebration. We haven't spoken yet, probably because they don't know what to say. I must admit, it is a bit awkward right now. One of them looks over and we make eye contact. I feel a little better on the inside.

I take another gulp of the margarita sweating in my hand and smile pretty. Perhaps if it's convincing enough, everyone will forget about the elephant in the room, finish their drinks, and leave. My husband, Jacob, is not here, and that's obvious since he was always the social one in the relationship. Only a handful of people know why he's absent, and I'm not ready to tell a soul more.

I thank Mike Michalowicz, one of my mentors, for his virtual attendance, right before I tease him for having the girliest glittered Zoom background.

"That's not a background. That's the wallpaper in my hotel room," he says in his Jersey accent. "You think *I* would have picked *this?*"

I tell him how his support means the world to me, and then we say our goodbyes.

I take a second to turn away from the camera and breathe. I don't like the attention.

AJ, my writing coach and one of the editors for my book, appears a couple of seconds later, but I don't see her. I am focused on the other people *in* the room, so her voice startles me. It's loud and clear and thick with emotion. "I'm so proud of you, Kasey," she says. "You've worked so hard."

Proud. I made her proud? The woman who taught me how to write, who pushed me, who helped me find my voice, who encouraged me to trust myself. She is proud of me? I nearly fumble my drink. I can't remember the last time I've heard those words. Have I *ever?*

Tears spring into my eyes, and I hastily blink to hold them in. *I'm not going to cry here, not in front of these people.* I take another large drink and feel the smooth burn as the alcohol slides down. Then I hear my Granny's voice in my head: *Kasey Renee, listen to her. She knows what she's a' talkin' bout. And lay off the booze, or I'll have to pray extra for ya come Sunday.*

"Well, thank you," I say finally, and try to arrange my face into the appropriate gracious expression. "You are a great teacher."

She laughs. "No, Kasey. Well, I mean, yes. I am. But *you* are a good writer. *You* wrote this book, and it's fantastic. *You* crossed the finish line. I just gave you a few tools. *You're* the star."

My throat tightens, and I know if I try to do more than smile and breathe, I will break down.

I don't feel like a star.

I feel like shit.

I have done everything I was supposed to do. I made mistakes, of course, but I went to college, got a degree, found a career, got married a couple of times, had some children, built a successful business, then built another, and another. I had money. I had respect. In some circles, I even had a little fame. I crossed every accomplishment, every event I wanted to go to, and every big purchase I'd been saving for off my bucket list. I bought a fucking hot tub just because I felt like it. And what did it get me?

A damn chlorine burn.

But I wrote something. I opened my heart and mind to my dream of authorship, poured myself onto the page, and today my first book baby is born. Amazon has been eagerly eating up preorders. I know because I've checked every five minutes. Today, finally, they will ship it to readers all over the world. People will hold my words in their hands, and their businesses will change.

I made my mentors proud. I made my teachers proud.

But I'm not proud.

In fact, I don't feel anything.

I'm numb.

Empty.

The moment I've been waiting for is here, but it feels just like any other day, just with more food in my kitchen and more people on my porch. I thought that after all my years of searching for things—success, accomplishments, love, respect—I would find the fulfillment. But I haven't.

It hasn't been in any of the places I've searched. Not in the relationships, not in the cities, not in the small towns, not in the power, and not in the success. It wasn't in my job, car, or dream house. It's not standing here in the middle of my friends and colleagues, listening to my mentors speak eloquently about how they knew I'd be great from the moment we met.

It's. Not. Here.

My life is not what it appears to others. My marriage is not what they think it is—at this point, I barely have a marriage at all. There's not much left other than a piece of paper that legally binds us to one another. There's no connection, no communication, and certainly no understanding or empathy.

I'm tired of pursuing success and still feeling empty inside, but they don't know that. I've kept it a secret from them, and probably myself, for a long time. But tonight, they're going to know—there's no way they couldn't. They'll probably think my lack of joy is about *him*, about Jacob not being here, but it's not. I'm not sad because of that. I'm rattled because of something else—something I'm not ready to tell anyone about yet.

The feelings take me back to a conversation with my first serious relationship, Frank, who eventually became my first husband, which happened nearly thirteen years ago when I was twenty-four years old.

"Go, Kasey," he said as our marriage was coming to an end. "Go find what you're looking for, whatever it is, because it's clearly not me. You're not satisfied, and I don't know that you'll ever be."

Those words have haunted me since the day he said them. They haunt me now as I stand here in a moment when I should be nothing *but* satisfied.

Maybe I am selfish.

I keep my smile fixed as I tell the rest of my virtual guests goodbye. Outside the sun has already set, and there are just a few red streaks in the sky as it fades into a deep midnight blue. Today is the day I officially became a published author and crossed the big to-do off my bucket list, and I feel like such a fraud. Faking a smile and pretending to be happy when I'm hiding so much from everyone.

No one knows that today would have been mine and Jacob's sixth wedding anniversary. Today is the day my attorney says my divorce petition is on the record, but no one knows that either. This is not the day, the life, or the feelings I ever imagined I would have.

Sitting with the few friends still hanging around, staring out over a beautiful view of Lake Cumberland, I realize, perhaps for the first time ever, nothing out here will ever satisfy me.

And that must mean that the answer I'm looking for is in *here*, in me—which is the most terrifying realization I've ever had.

The Morning After–July 20, 2021

Uncertainty, shame, and a smidge of relief linger thick in the air the morning after.

I wake to it, still sorting through the fog in my head, wondering if all of it is real. I pry my eyes open and give myself a moment before I swing my legs to the side of the bed to stand and stretch. As soon as my feet graze the floor, instinctively, almost like they know where I need to go, they take me back to the place I always gravitate toward: my porch, the reason I bought the house to begin with.

I fall into the corner cushion of the sectional I purchased as a housewarming gift. I cover my bare legs with the blanket I left out the night before and lay my head over on the armrest.

A deer strolls across the grass—must be a momma because three of her babies follow close behind. One stops for a moment to take a drink from the creek that runs through the front yard. Floating on the stubborn shards of green sprigs, my daughter's oversized yellow ball with pink polka dots is nudged between two trees. *I told her not to kick that thing down the hill.* The wind is light and brisk but nice on my cheeks, which still feel flushed.

I *try* to feel numb, but I can't. Usually, it's not this hard. I've been numb for years and I'm not anymore, but God, I want to be.

"You have an emotional hangover."

That's what Emily, my assistant, who also answers to "dearest friend," "publicist," "marketing coordinator," and an "all-around great human," would say. It was easier when I didn't feel things. It was easier when I was focused on getting shit done. Now, it's all about survival.

My thoughts race, and my heart feels like I've already had a couple of espressos, but I haven't. I think of everything from the bright green color of the leaves surrounding me to what I'm going to eat for lunch. *Maybe some leftover olives.*

I try to slow my mind so my heart will ease to a pitter patter, but the voice inside my head, the one that I barely recognize, keeps pressing. Negative thoughts, the catastrophizing ones, they flood any sense of normalcy that I hoped to have today.

I walk the porch, from one side to the other, taking deep breaths with every other step. *Inhale, exhale.* Then, the epiphany comes to me like the sun rising over the water every morning.

I'm good at avoiding anything painful; I think that's human nature. But for years, I told myself I talk myself *through* my feelings, but really, I just talk myself *out* of them. That's what I have been doing all these years—staying too busy to feel.

I don't have to do that anymore now that I know Jacob will be gone soon. I don't have to ignore my feelings to keep a marriage afloat. It has been my coping mechanism for pain. Now it's second nature, harder to stop than a big ole Smokey Mountain black bear rolling down a snow-covered hill.

Being numb to broken parent relationships, friendships, and loveships is the only way I've kept going. It has afforded me the space to do more work and move closer to my professional goals. I kept it tangible, concrete, and palpable. And that was easier.

Jacob never pressured me to share my feelings; he allowed me to stay in a window of tolerance that was familiar to me. For years, I fought my feelings hard. Heck, I was a therapist who had never gone to therapy, avoiding it with every fiber of my being. I earned a master's degree in mental health counseling, and in 2009 I immediately opened a private practice. It lasted long enough for me to see my first client, at which point I realized I needed more experience before I went out on my own. I spent the next several years learning and refining my skills, ultimately specializing in anxiety and panic disorders, and opening my own practice again for a second time in 2015.

I've always heard that we seek out careers that allow us to address and sort out the unresolved issues from our past. Maybe that's why I chose counseling. Maybe that's why I chose Frank, and later Jacob. Maybe that's how I ended up here.

———

When I was a kid, my Poppy called me strong, my Old Man called me focused, and now my colleagues call me successful, but I know what I really am. I am sensitive. Sitting here the morning after my book launch, recovering from a few too many bourbons and margaritas, feelings seem like all I have. I feel awake, I feel cold, I feel despair. I feel lonely, I feel robbed, I feel sad; it is all so overwhelming.

With every glance at my beautiful view, every look inward through the window behind me, I am reminded of the home that I worked so hard to buy but that never really felt the way I thought it would. I see the remnants of the night before sprinkled across my kitchen, and I notice an oversized vase of roses that was delivered at some point during the party. I must have been so busy entertaining my guests that I didn't even notice them.

I know exactly who they're from, though, and I haven't even read the card. *Jacob.*

I flash back to a time when the hypnotic smell of Granny's knockout roses drew me in through her front door. I used to stop and breathe them in, but now, I hold my breath.

Everything about *these* roses feels so obnoxious. I shake with anger thinking about all the flowers I walked in to see on my counter over the years given as a half-hearted apology—serving as a Band-Aid and a vessel for me to place my hurt, allowing me to sweep their withered and broken petals under the rug so that no one would see. That's what flowers from him have come to mean to me, and here I sit, looking at a swarm of them. Red and angry, like hornets ready to bite.

I should get up, throw them in the trash, and pretend this isn't happening.

The red stands out against the white marble countertops. I approach them like they could hurt me, with caution. I take a deep breath and tell myself it's okay to feel scared. It's okay to feel sad. It's okay to just feel.

"I'm proud of your milestone achievement. I hope you have fun with your friends."

I read it twice.

What. The. Hell?

My face illuminates in a crimson flush. I shake. My hands, trembling so bad I can't even bear to look at them, take on a mind of their own. To think about another form of passive aggressive manipulation any longer fills me full of rage. I reach down and pick up the vase with one hand, but it's heavier than I anticipate. Before I can secure it, it falls. The glass hits the side of the marble and shatters, scattering across the floor.

I walk over and grab the fancy trash can I bought when I moved in and bring it over to where I was first standing. Carefully, I drop to my knees to pick up the large shards of glass. The roses are spread across the hardwood floor. I save them for last.

It takes a couple of trips, but I retrieve the glass until there's nothing left but the flowers—just them and my feelings. Them and what's left of the life I thought I needed to finally feel joy.

These. Damn. Roses.

Why roses? Why not make an effort, instead? Why not changed behavior? Why did he choose to throw these in my face on the very day I was supposed to celebrate the very thing he watched me sacrifice everything for?

Tears stream down my face, but I don't want them to. I want them to stop. I want to run away. I want to leave and never come back, but I have kids. I have responsibilities. I have people who depend on me. I can't leave, and even if I could, I don't have anywhere to go.

On my knees, feeling the uncomfortable pain from the glass dust that in no way compares to the pain in my soul, I don't know what else to do to pass the moment, to distract from my feelings, besides count the damn things.

One, two, three, four. I throw them in the trash as I go.

More quickly after that. *Five, six, seven, eight . . .*

Nine, ten, eleven . . . twenty-one, twenty-two, twenty-three.

And they're gone.

In the trash, where they belong.

Sigh. It is the first full breath I take, until I realize something.

Wait.

I only count twenty-three roses: one short of two dozen. *Where is the last one?*

My body stops moving for a moment, maybe more, I don't know. Everything stops. My breath, my hearing, my ability to comprehend what is going on in this moment—in my life. I stand up and look around, giving my foyer one last glance before settling into the fact that there were only *twenty-three red roses.*

The missing one is nowhere to be found.

"Typical," I say instinctively.

No apologetic gesture could be complete without a subtle little hint, knowingly or not, that he would and could never give me everything. He would always withhold something, whether it be feelings or a flower, and there was nothing I could do to stop it.

Except stop it.

Therapy—July 2021

"You need therapy."

There it is. His parting shot.

As we stand in our bedroom a mere two days after the party, a couple of inches apart, we're as close as we've been to one another in months. We're arguing about another suitcase he packed so he could leave for good. I am exhausted.

So much has happened in the few short weeks leading up to this moment, I can't help but wonder if my life is ever going to be normal again. He accused me of cheating with a coworker, but there's more to it than that. I'm not cheating, but I did have a conversation with someone, and I can't tell him the details. It's their story to tell, not mine.

He does not agree.

When I wrote my book during the peak of the COVID-19 pandemic, I found myself isolated at home with him and the kids and a tremendous amount of fear about the future. The experience of writing a book during that time forced me to excavate feelings that I had buried for years. While trying to connect with my reader, I connected with myself for the first time in a long time. And it wasn't until then that I had the time and space to look around at my life, and I didn't like what I saw.

Hardened and calloused by that point, my heart's only function was to protect itself from pain. And with that rigidity came a lack of vulnerability. Jacob's and my lack of refuge in each other showed me that we had not cultivated safety in our relationship. My head should have rested on his shoulder each night to bring peace and calm, but it didn't. My words were not safe to share but used as weapons instead, and because of that, emotional safety could not exist. Because of that, *we* could not exist.

"I've been waiting for this," he says as he stuffs more clothes into the suitcase. His eyes are flat. Convinced of my infidelity, there's nothing in them but revenge.

Listening to his hatred, I see that the last ten years of our relationship have been nothing more than a house of cards. *Was he just using me? Was I just an opportunity for a better life? Did he only marry me because I was the mother of his child? Did he ever really love me?*

In the past I told myself that if I could just be patient, be forgiving, continue believing that the things that I acknowledged were wrong with our relationship were just "little," then the problems would go away, and I would be fine enough.

My body knew something hadn't been right all along. Just like the lights were turned on in the darkness I had been living, I think that maybe he *had* been waiting for this moment. I don't think he even liked me.

"I've been waiting for you to fuck up and now I'm going to ruin you. Your reputation. Everything you've built. I'll ruin everything you are, then I'll take everything you have. I know there's something going on with you and Kelsey," he says. "I saw you having lunch with her and drinking from the same straw. Looked pretty damn close to me."

"Can you just stop? Please. I'm not sleeping with her, Jacob, but you've accused me of it so much that I'm starting to consider it," I retaliate.

That was a lie. I wasn't "starting" to consider it—I had considered it before. Like the first time I ever spoke to her. But I couldn't share that with him—hell, I didn't even understand it myself. The closest I ever came to acknowledging the feeling was saying to him, "If something happens to you, I'll never be with another man again," because I wholeheartedly believed that.

With Jacob, I was in a constant state of high alert, but I thought that was normal. I'd seen that kind of dynamic play out my entire life between my mom and dad, my mom and stepdad, my sister and her ex-husband, my dad and stepmom, Granny and Poppy—everyone. I held my anxiety close because I didn't know what else to do with it—I certainly couldn't share it with him. My body told me to be careful in the relationship and always be on guard. My gut spoke to me louder than my heart did most of the time, but I chose to ignore it. I chose not to see the signs or connect any of the dots. It was easier that way. To turn the other cheek and pretend everything was fine.

I haven't told anyone about this because they all think we're happy. It would take hours to explain that I'm not. I know our divorce is going to come as a shock to people. It would take weeks to go through all the Little Things that led us here now, which don't seem so little, and I just don't have the energy.

Since I don't have a best friend to talk to, and I'm not close with my mom, I pull out my journal and start to write. I write down everything he told me, everything he did, everything I did, and what I said. I write it down mostly to understand, but I also want to remember. I never want to second-guess my decision to leave. I never want to repeat the same mistakes again with someone new. I never want him to make me think I'm leaving him for someone else. He'll never understand that the only person I'm leaving him for is *me*.

And that's the only reason I need.

The night after the book launch, still stewing over the roses in the trash and how numb I felt after the launch, I replay Jacob's words over and over in my head. "You need therapy."

I belt out a scream, as loud as my voice will carry. My entire body shakes with the force of it. When I exhaust myself, when every muscle in my being trembles from the pain, and my cry finally ends in a slow sob, I let my head fall between my knees and rest my cheek against the cool tile floor.

Therapy might not be a bad idea, I tell myself. Going to therapy just means that I am strong enough to ask for help and willing to share my life's stories with a stranger. The feelings that came along with the book launch showed me that fulfillment was something I would only find by turning inward.

Now is the time to redirect the search that I have put off for so long.

I can't run anymore.

I remember something that my friend Tara once told me. We sat on the phone, several states apart, but it felt like we were sitting side by side drinking a glass of wine.

"Here's the thing about fear, Kasey. It's counterintuitive. Wanna know why?"

She didn't even give me an opportunity to answer her question. That's her way. She talks like she's letting you inside her brain. Every single thought comes out of her mouth. In that way, she's fearless. In that way, she's trustworthy.

"I'll tell you why. If we fear something, we must know where it is at all times. We must keep it close. We think we're avoiding it, but the only way to do that is to know exactly where it is. Which means it's right there with us *always*. We think we're running from it, but we're not. We're running into it and *pretending* we're not."

It's not until I recall this conversation that I realize the only way to truly find what I'm looking for is to first recognize what I'm running from.

It's like a light comes on in the basement of my heart. Bugs skitter away, but I've seen them, and I know they're there. They are fears I've pushed down and pushed down and pretended I didn't know about for years. I can see them now. And I need to expose them if I'm ever going to be free. The fearless, adventurous little girl that I used to be deserves that. *I* deserve that. I need to do it for her if I won't do it for anything or anyone else. I need to do it for my future, for my kids and *their* future.

Jacob was right. I do need to go to therapy, not for his sake but for mine.

Fear–September 2021

"On a scale from one to ten, how much do you love yourself?" the therapist asks. *Well, you don't waste any time.*

It's the first actual session we've had together aside from the brief phone consultation a week prior. I found her online when I didn't think I could sit in or sort through my feelings alone any longer.

Now, I'm staring nervously at my computer screen, in the direction of a woman who looks to be about the same age as me. Her website says she specializes in "professional women going through a divorce."

Let's see . . . how do I tell this lady that on the outside, I pretty well have my shit together, but on the inside, I'm a basket-case nutjob who doesn't know if she's coming or going? How do I tell her that I'm here getting therapy because I realize I hate my life; I have no emotions other than anger; I don't like sex; the only thing that gets me though the day is thinking about going to sleep; my husband thinks I'm cheating on him; and, if I wasn't so self-conscious about my body, I'd be seriously considering it?

Clearly, "professional woman going through a divorce" is not all I am and that's not all that's wrong with me, but it seems the most appropriate description of my problems, so I feel reassured that I chose the right therapist.

She speaks kindly—softly. I'm intimidated, but I try to hide it with a smile.

Immediately, I'm caught off guard by her question about self-love. I was expecting a little small talk first—maybe we can discuss the incessant rain or the fact that there has been a massive storm system blowin' up the East Coast this week—but no, she hits me where it hurts in the first sixty seconds.

Relax. It's a standard question for an intake, one she probably asks all her clients to establish a baseline, but I'm not them. It feels way too personal for me.

I've never considered the concept of loving myself. I don't know what *that* is.

I question my own credibility, especially since I'm a therapist, too.

How'd I miss it all these years? Did anyone ever teach me to love myself? I don't think so.

I am extremely uncomfortable. I want to be anywhere but here. I want to feel anything but this. What does self-love have to do with me needing therapy anyway? I'm just trying to get through a divorce; I'm trying to get rid of the night terrors, panic attacks, and all the little things that trigger them. I'm trying to release the shame of another failure. How does loving myself help me do any of those things?

I don't know how *self-love* is going to help me move past the pain I feel. It doesn't make my situation any easier right now. It doesn't remove the weight that's been sitting on my chest since the weeks leading up to the party.

In my years of clinical training, I saw many clients just like me who told themselves their problem was unique. But that's the problem. We think we live and create bad habits in isolation, but we don't. Others experience the same things, and I'm sure this therapist knows that.

We have an inherent ability to love ourselves and without whipping out my textbooks on Attachment Theory and Internal Family Systems, I know that our ability to do this comes from how we've received it from others, especially in childhood. Those of us who have experienced unmet needs, anxious or dismissive parents, or abuse and/or emotional neglect can be left feeling like they're failing or that there is something wrong with *them*.

That's me.

My own family didn't know how to meet my emotional needs and never have, so for years I searched for a replacement. The time I spent trying to belong to the families I married into left me feeling even more isolated. I didn't know how to open up and fully allow them into my life, so they never really became a part of it. Sensing my resistance, they shut me out even more, leaving me feeling like an outsider.

I understand loving yourself on an intellectual level. I know what love is, technically, but emotionally? How does it feel? I don't know.

I sit staring blankly, thinking, and I haven't said one word.

I bet she thinks I'm crazy. A shitty therapist. Dissociative. Hell, I don't know.

I try my darndest to get my wits about me. I quickly consider rattling something off to move the moment forward, but I don't. I want my response to be honest, genuine, and thoughtful, even if it does make me look stupid. If it makes the panic stop long enough for me to sleep through the night, any amount of humiliation will be worth it.

Do the work. Trust the work. Right?

Maybe there is an answer in me somewhere, but I can't seem to find it. I take my time because she does not rush me, but secretly, I hope she will become distracted so I can avoid the question altogether. The awkward silence doesn't faze her. She is not letting me off the hook.

She's good.

"I don't even know what that looks like," I finally say. I look down at the keyboard when I make this admission, because I'm embarrassed.

I'm struggling. Like knee-high muck boots struggling. Like trying to take one foot out of the muddy water, just to put the other one right back in. I move slowly. It hurts. I use muscles I don't know I have. I'm wet. I'm heavy. I'm uncomfortable. I'm a fish out of water, but I'm not lost because she's there, and that gives me hope. This may be the first time we've met, but I can tell she knows what she's doing. She's done this before, perhaps even for herself.

She remains quiet.

Now a quarter of the way into this session, I can't fathom self-love, but I see that I need to try. It's the first question she asked me, the only one so far. My situation is her specialty so there must be a reason that this is the baseline she wants to gather. I trust her process and tell myself to push through. I need to get better. This will help.

"I've never seen it, felt it, or experienced it in any way."

No wonder I feel lost in this question. No wonder I feel like I'm wading in murky waters. Because in a lot of ways, I am—and I have been for most of my life.

"I'm thinking about what it looks like to love someone. I respect them. I genuinely care about their feelings, well-being, and everything that makes them who they are. Is loving yourself the same?" I ask.

I really don't know the answer.

"Think about the truest, most genuine, most unconditional love you've ever felt," she says.

It's not my parents or my ex. It must be my kids.

I love them for who they are, regardless of their flaws. I forgive them for their bad behaviors, and I see their hearts. I love my kids unconditionally.

"Well, that is most certainly *not* how I feel about myself," I say.

"How *do* you feel about yourself?"

"I don't think I feel any sort of way."

I guess this is what happens when you use numbness to survive.

I start to see how repressing my feelings got me where I am now, but in other ways, it helped me. Numbness helped me avoid pain and dig myself out of bankruptcy, kept me from being homeless, and allowed me to focus solely on building my future with financial security. It helped me get to a place where I could be proud of my accomplishments and my growth as a female entrepreneur in a small town where that's never expected or respected, for that matter. My grit allowed me to persevere even when I wanted to quit. My determination made me a force to be reckoned with in the healthcare and coaching industry.

Wait.

"You know, I'm confident in what I *do*, but not *who* I am," I say aloud.

"Interesting. Then tell me more about *who* you are."

I don't know the answer to this, either. I mean, I am a mom. I am a business owner. I *was* a wife. That part's easy, but in a lot of ways those are also things I *do*.

Maybe I can't describe this because I've let what I do define me. Maybe because I don't know what self-love is. It makes sense. How could I love someone I don't know? I certainly don't treat myself like I treat my children, and they are the only true representation of love that I have.

I'm critical of my looks, my work ethic, and my ability to lead. I judge myself for my shortcomings and often tell myself I'm not doing enough, so I try to do more. It's never enough. That leaves me feeling perpetually defeated. It's disheartening. I would never do that to my children. So why do I do it to myself?

I start to break down. I feel it in my stomach first, then it moves up into my chest. I try to swallow to distract my eyes from the tears that are about to leak out from the inner corners.

Don't do it. Don't do it. Don't let her see you cry. I hold them in tight.

I was never allowed to cry. I was told to cry in my room, dry it up, suck it up. Crying was weakness, crying was for babies, crying got you nowhere. Crying got *me* nowhere so I told myself to stop. Pointless. It won't do me any good.

"What are you feeling in your body right now?" she asks me.

That's all it took for me to break.

No one has ever asked me how I feel.

"I don't know."

I don't know how to *feel* in my body. *Sad* is the only word that comes to mind. All I can feel are the tears that are streaming down my face.

I think about my children for all of thirty seconds, and I can't help but see myself as a little girl again. Tall, lanky, and tan in the summer, playing in the trees at Poppy and Granny's house. Golden brown freckles on my face, curly chestnut hair, and a little upturned nose. I have very few memories before the age of six. But even then, I don't remember being told *I love you,* except by Granny. I remember how uncomfortable it made me feel, how unnatural it was.

I recall snapshots from when I was sixteen, too afraid to disturb my stepdad to walk down the metal spiral staircase from my bedroom loft and pee, so terrified that he'd wake up and my mom would be annoyed, that I'd hold it. I did this so often that I had chronic UTIs and eventually had to take daily medication to mitigate the problem.

I think about the times when holding it was not even an option, so I'd open my bedroom door, walk out on the little princess balcony, and let it roll off the roof. I believed that was the best option: avoiding the "hard" conversation with my mom about how I sometimes needed to pee at night.

I think about my grandparents and how their house was the only place I ever received affection, even if it was a pinch on the butt or a messy head rub. I think about how I felt shipped from one place to another based on whether my behavior was good or not, how sometimes I felt like a business transaction. I remember often feeling ignored and disregarded. I only knew the secret kind of love, the love they kept inside, unexpressed—the kind that my parents probably felt but didn't know how to show me.

"At some point I started to believe that my needs didn't matter much," I say.

Her expression changes. I see her face soften. Some of my childhood experiences were not okay. I'm only starting to realize it as I speak it aloud.

"When we're taught from an early age that our feelings don't matter, we learn not to have any," she says.

Damn.

Yes, I can see that. I didn't feel anything but anger and hadn't for a long time. This is why.

No wonder I can't answer her question, the one that should have taken two seconds to resolve, but here we are, still in purgatory.

This is what I need, someone to help guide me through my feelings again so that I can process the memories, even if it is painful. I need to take ownership, and then learn who I am, because I no longer know.

"I don't think I have a framework to know what self-love looks like," I say. "I don't even think I know what *love* looks like."

I never had a foundation for understanding unconditional love, and certainly have no idea what it feels like. My past has given me only small glimpses of it, conditional on things like doing good, pleasing others, and living up to their expectations of me.

No wonder I don't understand.

No wonder I am sad.

No wonder I have felt the need to search for something in all the wrong ways.

No wonder I haven't looked inward.

I stall. No one I know is a model for self-love; in fact, all I've ever seen is self-deprecation and destruction, not love, grace, or respect. I begin to talk more about my family, how I grew up, and without intention, the words slip out.

"Most of the time I still don't feel like anyone loves me."

I stop as soon as the words leave my mouth.

I can't believe I just said that.

My chest thumps, and it hurts with each breath I take. I bite my bottom lip and start to pick at my thumbnail. My hands go numb, and I can't make myself look at her. I don't want to see someone else's pity. I never have. I'm ashamed to admit this; it feels like it's my fault that either no one loves me or that I feel like they don't.

She interrupts my thoughts that could have continued for quite some time.

"What are you afraid of, Kasey?"

I avoid the question with a question, "What kind of fear are you—" but she stops me. "Kasey," she pauses with authority, "what are you afraid of?"

I blurt it out, almost in a fit of anger. "Unlovable. I'm afraid I'm unlovable, okay."

There. I said it.

From Two to Portugal–
September 2021

It takes me until the last ten minutes of our first session to finally answer my therapist's question.

"Look. I don't like to fail. In fact, I hate it. F'n *hate* it. But I know that when I do, it makes me stronger. What I'm about to tell you, I know you're going to write down and I know you're going to ask me about every session, so I need you to understand that this is hard for me."

"It's okay. I know it's hard," she says.

"I love myself a *two*, and that's being generous," I say. "I want to love myself a ten. I need that so I can be the person I want to be. I don't want to run from fear anymore."

This admission feels good—kind of like puking up poison, it hurts in the moment, but I know it will save my life. I'm incredibly vulnerable, perhaps the most exposed I have ever felt. I am uncomfortable to the point of no return. I can't go back now. I can't change my mind. I can't unsay it. Expel the bad. Replace with good.

It's a *two*.

I'm afraid of failure, but I've kept the fear of it so close. Failing means I'm not enough. Not being enough would mean no one would want me. If no one wants me, I'll be alone. If I'm alone, my greatest fear is confirmed: I'm unlovable.

I see it all so clearly now.

Every time I failed, someone left. Small failure or big, it didn't matter. So I lived in a constant state of fearing abandonment. The potential of another failure easily sent me spiraling. Like if I rolled my eyes rather than nodding respectfully, if I expressed my opinion about excessive amounts of Red Bull and cigarettes one consumed, if I showed up later than someone believed I should, they threatened to leave me.

When I dated someone of the wrong race, caused a ruckus around town, didn't go to church every Sunday, someone was "done" with me. Now, I connect the two—I associate failure with being alone. That's why I stayed in toxic relationships when my body told me to run. That's why I forced myself to hustle and grind in businesses that were not serving me. That's why I forgot what joy was.

"So, what are we going to do about it?" I ask.

"Well, *you* will recognize your fears, learn from your failures, and then you're going to believe you are enough. You're going to trust yourself enough to love yourself again. And your life is going to change," she says.

I let that sink in.

I'm going to LEARN to love myself. Okay. I know that process; I taught it to people for years when I was practicing, just not to myself, apparently.

I feel a little more confident now. This feels more familiar.

"Okay. I will commit to trying," I tell her.

I know I can do anything I put my mind to, but that has been my problem for a long time. I haven't put my mind to anything like this. I've run from it, but I know I can't do that anymore.

"Oh, and most importantly," she adds, "I want you to plan a celebration."

"Huh? For what?" There's nothing to celebrate.

"A year from now, when you love yourself, your life is going to be different. I want you to plan something to honor this achievement."

"You mean before it actually happens?"

"Yes, because *it's going to happen.*"

"Okay, then. I'm going to Portugal!"

It bursts out of me before I can second-guess it. That beautiful country with limestone cliffs overlooking the Atlantic Ocean, the history, the culture, the surfing, the music festivals, and the Portuguese people who are known to be kind, open, and sincere—that's where I want to be. It's been a dream I've kept silent, quietly growing in my heart with every slamming door, crying child, judging stare, and Unisom tablet. Maybe, if this therapist lady is right and I can learn to love myself, my life will be different.

So I am going to love myself. And to do that I'm going to learn about myself. Then I'm going to be patient, extend grace, and understand myself as a messy work in progress. It's going to be hard, and I know that. But when it's done—*Portugal.*

Feelings—Late September 2021

Dear Journal,

My therapist told me to journal how I feel. This is how I feel.

Not quite as shit-like as the morning after my party, so that's good. It's more of an ache now. I realize I want a relationship one day that is deep and strong.

But I haven't been honest with myself about some things, and I've been keeping secrets from everyone, and it's eating away at me.

I don't know when it started, and right now I don't even know how to put it into words. What comes to mind is guilt.

Yeah, guilt.

I feel guilty for wanting more. For thinking there might be something better for me, something different. I feel guilty for even considering putting my needs first.

On days like today, I can't help but ask myself if *this is all there is?* I want to feel full of life, but I don't.

I've spent years looking for something that fulfills me—my mind, body, and soul. And I'm tired of coming up short.

I thought doing more would do it. But it hasn't. Instead of doing more, I think I need to do something different.

~Guilt

For You (#IAmHere)

Dear Reader,

Here's the thing: I'm not a physical kind of runner, and up until this point in my life I didn't know there was any other type. But there is. There's a fleeing discomfort kind of runner—the kind who uses subject changes, humor, and deflection (and when worse comes to worst, sometimes even sprinting to hide in the bathroom) to avoid the emotions that make you want to dig yourself into a hole and never come out again. But I did it for twenty years until I realized I was just calling it something else because that made it easier: I called it ambition, determination, chasing dreams—I called it searching.

It showed up in my quest to find myself by running off to Chicago at nineteen, and when I came back home and became a teacher. It showed up in my desire to become an entrepreneur, and in the many ways I pushed myself. It showed up in my relationships, in my two failed marriages, and in my dysfunctional family. Now it's obvious that I was doing more than just searching, but I didn't realize it at the time.

Even after I became a licensed professional counselor at twenty-six, and even after a decade of experience with clients, I didn't see it. I was blind to my own emotions. I didn't understand the meaning behind my own behaviors. I thought I wanted to be successful, respectable, and to be taken seriously. For years I believed that searching for more would get me closer to happiness, but it never did.

It wasn't until I stood there at my book launch among friends that I realized I had achieved everything I worked for all those years, and I felt no different. I thought, if all of "that" can't make me happy, then what can?

Change.

It *would* take change. It *will* take change.

I don't surround myself with people who will challenge me, listen to me, or validate me. I surround myself with people who support *what I do*, but not *who I am*.

And that is the problem.

For years I let shiny objects guide my search. From that came five businesses, two of which were multi-million-dollar ones, and one was pretty darn close. Shiny objects gave me something to look forward to, something to focus on, something to work toward, but I am still running.

I don't know what your search looks like, but I imagine it mirrors my experience in some way. If you feel dissatisfied, if you wonder that you might be settling, if you feel like you're spinning your wheels lacking purpose, you could be searching. If you find yourself filling a void with "things," you might be searching. Or maybe you're like me, and you're not *just* searching; maybe you're running, too. And if you are, the only way to find what you're searching for is to recognize what it is you're running from.

Let that sink in.

The only way to know what you're searching for is to first recognize what you're running from.

So that's where we must start.

Fear.

We run from what scares us.

What scares us is probably what we need the most.

I'll be here to remind you that you can do scary things. You *can* do this. *We* can do this together. I would never ask you to do something I wouldn't do myself, which is why I structured this book the way I did. I'll take you through my process, doing it first, allowing you to read my stories and my journal entries, and then I'll explain it so you can do something similar. I will share my reflections, the lessons I learned, and then I'll give you instructions to try it yourself.

What follows is the path I took to rediscover myself and my joy—something I hadn't felt since I was a girl. My hope is that by sharing that path with you, you can then embark on a similar journey.

1. **Remember (Inner Child).** It starts there. Remembering who you once were, your Inner Child: what she loved, what lit her up, what sparked curiosity, because that is where joy is found.

2. **Awareness (Big Things).** What happened in your life to bring you to this point? Who are you now? This is how we grow—we must first know where joy is *not*.

3. **Understanding (Little Things).** These are the little details that give your life meaning. Your life is not just a series of random events. When you understand how the Big Things and the Little Things affect you, you can move forward with confidence.

4. **Change.** Awareness and understanding bring about change. When we choose joy, it affects our habits, our hobbies, and how we spend our energy, ultimately affecting the quality of our life.

5. **Choosing Joy.** Because it lights us up. It takes every moment of life and brings forth an opportunity for feeling. **This is the end step, the goal of everything.**

Through my stories, through the practical applications you will find in these letters For You, and through the unfiltered rawness of my journal entries, you will find the path toward your own personal fulfillment. It may not look exactly like mine, and that's okay. Your journey is your own.

Give it a try.

Your Back Porch Bestie,

K

P.S. Just so you know, I'm calling you a Seeker because you chose this book, and since you're obviously reading it, it might mean that you feel like something is missing in your own life; you just may not have realized it until now. You're searching for something, so you're one of us now.

P.S.S. Oh yeah, you might want a dedicated notebook or stapled scraps of paper to see you through this process. Me? I used an oversized blue notebook. It doesn't have to be anything fancy, just something to draw out your life on—maybe with enough space to jot a few feelings here and there. Grab yourself something to write on, slap your name on it, and let's get this party started.

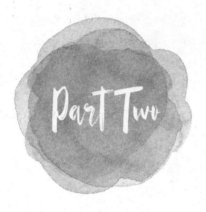

Remember

YOUR INNER CHILD

• Who is the little girl that lives inside of you? •

"I couldn't heal because I kept
pretending I wasn't hurt."
~unknown

The wounds of our Inner Child may not be made by our own hand, but they are within our power to heal. Those hurts may have put us in survival mode, where we are hypersensitive to the moods of others, afraid to settle, afraid to trust, and afraid to let joy in. Changing that response starts with Remembering what happened to us.

The Work—October 2021

I sit with my therapist again, ready to do the work she told me was coming in our first session. I am ready to Remember. I am ready to dig deeper into who Kasey, the little girl, was, what she needed, and what she once loved. Until I understand *her*, I'll never understand *me*.

"Who played an important role in your childhood?" she asks.

"My mom and dad, of course. Other than that, I spent most of my time at Poppy and Granny's."

"Tell me about that," she says.

I prepare myself for the memories and the feelings that must be sorted through, ones I haven't looked for in years—the people who made an impact on my childhood. The good times and the bad, what I wish I could forget, what I have been reluctant to think about, so many things I must process.

That starts with allowing myself to Remember.

The people, the things, *the fear.* I haven't talked about my past much because no one has ever asked me. I try not to think about it because some parts make me sad. Not just because there were some hurts, but because I miss life as a carefree little girl.

The simplicity.

The freedom.

The joy.

Mom—Summer 1995

I'm nine years old in my first concrete memory with my mom. I sit shotgun on the tattered bench seat of a 1984 Oldsmobile Cutlass that basically resembles a beat-up land boat. Swallowed by a grayish-blue cloth interior, the fabric is torn in several places, and a pop of orange foam sticks out from underneath.

The thick stench of cigarette smoke and Estée Lauder perfume penetrate every stitch of my tank top and cloth shorts. Mom's car reeks of sadness and grief, and it's stained with years' worth of tears. I don't understand why, but it is obvious she is not happy. She is hurting.

She sits beside me silently gazing out the window, thinking about who knows what. I look over sneakily every so often to check her body language, as she takes the backroads to the house of Granny, Dad's mom. It is a Friday, and I am ready to spend my weekend roaming around my grandparents' property, spying on Poppy, going for rides with the Old Man, and sewing throw pillows with Granny in the garage.

Puffing on a Marlboro Light, Mom drives with one hand on the wheel and the other on the window's ledge. The window is cracked just enough to draw out the smoke, and I pray that if I hold my breath, I won't end up with lung cancer one day.

No makeup again. Her permed hair with frosted tips is slung back in a white banana clip. I don't remember the last time she curled and teased it up like she used to. She's probably had another fight with my dad and doesn't have the energy to do herself up real nice today. They both want a divorce, but money seems to be getting in the way of finalizing it. The three jobs Mom works is barely enough to keep us afloat, let alone pay legal fees.

I reach to turn on the radio as we pass by the Grand Central Shopping Center, the most popular place in my town for teenagers to cruise. The faint sound of "Whoomp! (There It Is)" plays. Without a second thought, I reach my hand back across the front seat to turn up the volume.

We aren't much of a music family; we aren't much of a "noise" kind of family, but I've heard this song on the stereo system I got for my ninth birthday, and I'm dying to hear it again.

"Turn off the music," Mom says sternly. The way her piercing eyes look at me when she gives an order causes the chicken skin to rise on my forearms. All her kids know that when Mom tells you to do something, you best do it, and you best do it fast.

"But I like this song."

"Yeah, and I like the peace and quiet, but that doesn't seem to matter to you much right now."

Matter to me? Everything matters to me.

I notice everything important to her. I leave her alone in her bedroom when she tells me she's depressed. I bring her crackers when she says she hasn't eaten all day. I check back several times only to see them in the same place I put them. I play outside until the sun goes down when she "just wants to be alone." I stay in my room reading books, escaping into a world where people listen when I speak and care about what I have to say. I nestle into my yellow pleather beanbag dreaming about writing one of my own someday. For once, I want to be in control of the story. I want to choose the ending.

Her instinctive, quick demand unsettles me, but it's not much different than any other day, honestly.

"I said: Turn. Off. The. Music."

So I do. Sinking down into the seat as deep as my little body can, I become quiet and tell myself to dissolve—*pretend like you're invisible, Kasey.*

"We're here," she says as she pulls into the driveway. Her tone has the finality of a "goodbye" and the bite of a "get out."

She probably just needs some time to herself.

I mumble something like a "see ya" as I fling myself out of the passenger door with the squeaky handle, and into the cool, perfectly maintained grass of Poppy's yard—the place I can be as loud as I want to be.

Two steps away, I feel a tug in my stomach, like when I sneak an extra cookie between meals or when I catch Mom crying after she thinks I've gone to sleep. I turn around to wave one last time, feeling a little sad about leaving her, but she is already backing out of the driveway, her head turned the other way.

———

"Sounds like your mom had a lot riding on her shoulders?" my therapist says.

I nod. That was an understatement. Mom got primary custody of me in the divorce, and Dad saw me every other weekend. It was a loose visitation schedule; I came and went as I pleased. I ended up spending more time with Granny and Poppy than anyone else.

Mom used to say that she knew she wasn't the "fun" parent, but I could count on her for everything I needed. From school clothes to sports equipment, I knew she'd take care of it. She worked as many jobs as it took to make ends meet. She probably felt like she gave so much to everyone else that she didn't have much left for herself.

Kind of like she'd lost herself, too.

"I guess that's why she was so tired. And so depressed," I say.

She worked her fingers to the bone at the sewing factory, put her best face forward at the local Tumbleweed restaurant, and worked the cash register at Lowes just to make sure I had everything I needed. I don't know many people who would work that hard for someone else, but Mom did.

"What was her childhood like?" my therapist asks.

She didn't talk to me about it much. I pieced together some of the stories she told me, like the one where she walked a long distance to school and got chased and pecked to near death by a slew of chickens. I know they were poor and grew up in a tiny farmhouse out in the country. Her bedroom was upstairs in a loft that she shared with her four sisters. She told me how hard her mom, Lillie, worked, and how much pride she took in making sure that every child, back then, and in the years that followed, always had a Christmas gift. She told me about her daddy, who was quite a drinker and not nice to her momma but took a liking to her more than his other kids, and how that made her feel.

Special. But obligated to make sure he was taken care of. She felt like she had to protect him.

"I think they had a special kind of bond, different than the rest of the sisters."

"Was *her* momma affectionate with her?" the therapist asks.

"I don't think so."

My Granny Lillie wasn't much of a hugger, kisser, or a tell-you-she-loves-you kinda lady; she was more of the strong, silent, and stoic type. I never saw her cry. I never heard her complain. As a triplet, she, her brother Willie, and sister Zillie grew up during the depression in a family full of youngins. It had to be tough to live back then. She handed down that toughness, strong will, and work ethic to my mom, and I guess that's where I got it from.

"Your Granny Lillie was probably raised to be independent," my therapist says. "And passed that style of parenting along to your mom."

There wasn't much time or energy left back then to worry about one's mental health when tobacco needed to be harvested, animals had to be fed, and a garden required tending to. Keeping the kids alive was an accomplishment in and of itself.

"Mom took care of all my physical needs, but not my emotional ones," I say. "I don't ever remember her telling me she loved me." I'm not sure if she knew how.

This comes out of nowhere. I have never told anyone, at least not until now. Mom *showed* me she loved me by caring for me, but I didn't feel attached to her in the same way I do to my own children. She wasn't my comfort, my safe place—no one was. She didn't feel like home, and I always wanted that.

She had a serious way about her, one that I know she got from her mom, my Granny Lillie. I can see that I have been a lot like that for the last ten years. Mom was afraid to be alone, even though she would have never said that out loud, and as much as I hate to admit it, I think have been, too. She always looked for the negative, which I viewed as being a realist. But it's not being a realist; it's a joy thief. Along with all the memories, I can see more and more how I've been slowly evolving into her.

"That must have hurt, not having that kind of safety and comfort. I think your Inner Child is wounded, Kasey."

"So this is what that looks like—*I* am what that looks like? A wounded Inner Child?"

She nods and smiles a little.

"Mom's Inner Child is probably wounded, too," I say.

"Yeah, it can be generational," she says.

Mom didn't go to therapy, so she wouldn't have known that. She would not have known how to heal. It makes a little more sense now as to why I had such a hard time adjusting to motherhood when I had Maime. I felt love for her, but it was strange the first time I said the words. It had never been modeled for me. All I had to go on was instinct and what I thought I "should" do, what I should feel, how I should act.

It still feels that way sometimes, if I'm being honest.

"Did any of your caregivers tell you they loved you regularly?" she asks.

"Yes. Just my Granny."

Big Granny–Summer 1995

"Granny, where did I come from?" I ask as I reach down to pluck the plumpest strawberry from the vine. I give it a quick blow to get rid of most of the dirt and pop it straight into my mouth, pulling out the stem and chucking it into the surrounding grass. "And don't start with that cabbage patch stuff!"

For as long as I can remember, everyone insisted they found me in a cabbage patch, curled up, sleeping under a soft leaf, just waiting to be picked and brought home to be part of *their* family. At the ripe old age of nine, I know that none of my friends' parents found *them* in the garden, so I highly doubt I come from one either.

Big Granny, whose real name is Sylvia, my dad's mom, is the last holdout, still insisting if I'd let her that maybe I just naturally sprung up in her garden one day.

"What'ya means, where'd you come from?" she says, wiping sweat off her brow. Her poufy silver hair stands as high on her head as she is able to tease and spray in place with the hairspray in the purple can, but it offered no shade and was beginning to droop over slightly in the heat of a humid Kentucky summer. Carefully styled high and arched, her thin little eyebrows match the intensity of her hair. She opens her eyes just enough to see me frowning back at her. At that moment, she *and* her eyebrows are fully curious but also slightly concerned about where this conversation might go.

I give her my best shrewd glare and wait for the real answer, just out of reach from any swatting hands.

She sighs and gives in with reluctance. "You're a Mitchell, Kasey Renee. You came from *yourn* momma and *yourn* daddy." Her bright lilac lipstick is extra noticeable and glimmers under the sun, making her thin lips look iced over. Her brassiere (that's what she calls it) hangs out the side of her two-sizes-too-big cutoff T-shirt.

"You got your momma's attitude, your daddy's temper, your Poppy's smarts, and well, you got the rest from me, Sugar Foot."

I guess that makes a little sense. I can see some of those similarities in each of them. Mom is strong. Dad is patient with me, but I see how easily he becomes angry with my brother, who is fourteen years older than me and out of the house already. My sister is a year younger than him and doesn't live at home either. Poppy is smart and methodical but kind of scary. And Granny, well, she is quirky and fun.

She has a way of drawing a crowd and keeping them captivated by her stories. Whether she's with me and all my friends, or gossiping with the old biddies at church, she is Mrs. Center of Attention. Here, among the vines, stalks, and squash blossoms, somehow, she demands my full attention, too.

"Ya sure?" I say as I cock my head to the side, and a little strawberry juice drops on to my white tank top.

"I reckon I am. Come on," she says as she walks away, waving her arm as if to herd me back to the house.

"Ya hungry? I'll make you a ham salad sammich." Her voice becomes fainter the farther she moves away. That is her way. When I ask something hard, she leaves, distracts me, or offers something to eat.

I stand there in the garden amidst the watermelons and radishes, feeling comfort from the very things she grew with her hands and the dirt she worked so hard to nourish. There *is* a connection to her, a grounding of sorts. Maybe she did find me here because it does kind of feel like home.

She wobbles away, in the purple polyester pants she wears nearly every day she works in the garden, stocking feet and all. I think about her and how we're alike more than different. Her wit, her charm, her sass, her love for creating things—I see it. I see her inability to sit still, her desire to be a little mischievous, and how she never lets anything go to waste. I am a lot like that, too.

I wait until she's past the freshly tilled dirt and reaches the gravel driveway. She hops around like a cat on coal as she moves across. Stocking feet aren't meant for rocks any more than for the garden's soil. Just a few more steps and she'll be inside the garage where the Ford Fairmont my Poppy bought her is parked. She calls her Black Beauty.

It's funny how I always know what she is about to do before she does it—the connection we have, and how much I pay attention to her mannerisms. It seems like magic to my kid-mind; I've seen this song and dance too many times not to believe it.

Ham salad with salt and fresh cracked black pepper is Big Granny's famous midday sandwich with a secret recipe that isn't so secret. We all know the mystery ingredient is whatever is old and out of date from the refrigerator, even if it is a hotdog or something else just as nasty, but somehow, the sandwich always makes me feel better.

I wait long enough for her to be out of eyesight before I take my first step out of the garden. I don't think I want to help her cook today. I stare at my maple tree instead. The one that sits strong overlooking Poppy and Granny's garden. My thoughts travel everywhere but inside the house for a ham salad sandwich. I have something else on my mind.

—————

"That's a lot for a nine-year-old little girl to be holding on to," my therapist says. "What was it that you had on your mind?"

I was curious. Always full of questions, searching for answers, for meaning. I was never satisfied until I got the whole story—until it made complete sense.

"I felt something that day—out of place a little bit," I say. "I was trying to find where I belonged, and something told me I wasn't born into the Mitchells."

I was conflicted. I knew I was different. Yeah, I looked a little like my Old Man, but I wanted things that he didn't. I accepted things that he couldn't accept. I liked to dream, think about what I would be when I grew up, where I would live, what kind of career I would have. Poppy said I had no business being anywhere but on Slate Branch Road. Plus, I am the only one in the family with green eyes.

I knew that some things weren't safe to talk about—so I didn't, but it pained me. Other times, I couldn't resist. Like that time in the pew of my Southern Baptist church, I wrote notes in the margins of the bulletin to ask my Granny Sylvia over Sunday supper.

"But Granny, why does the Bible say to love, but people in the church fight so much?" She didn't like these questions.

"Hey, Granny, why does everyone in the church have pink skin? Why can't my friend Sheena from Grand Central Apartments come to church with us? Is it because her skin isn't pink?"

She *really* didn't like this question.

"But Granny, why can't I marry someone like Sheena? Would God still love me? Would *you* still love me?"

She ignored me most times, paying me nary a bit of mind.

"Don't ask questions when it comes to Jesus, Kasey Renee. All you need to worry about is gettin' to heaven."

"But . . ."

"God wants men to be with women—pink skin to be with pink skin, brown skin to be with brown skin—we're not supposed to mix," Granny says.

"I don't see why that matters at all," I say.

"Quiet before your Poppy hears you talkin' nonsense!"

I never understood. Why can't I question the Bible? Why can't I doubt Poppy or Dad? Or the preacher? What's wrong with trying to understand? What's wrong with forming my own opinion? From the time I was old enough to establish self-awareness, I always felt like I was different. I haven't always felt like that was okay.

I don't want to be closed off and closed-minded. I don't want to live by rules I don't understand or believe in like they do. I don't need to have babies that look and act just like me when I could adopt and have a family that is blended and unordinary. I like the colors of freedom. I like interesting. I like different. And my family didn't.

"It sounds like you had a good idea of what your life would look like at a pretty early age. Do you think it turned out like that?" my therapist asks.

"No."

I wanted a house full of kids. I didn't know how to get them, but they'd be mine. I wanted a life full of fun and laughter, and that's not what mine has been like. I wanted to lie down to sleep each night with someone who loved me as a human being above all else. I wanted someone who loved me for me, not just because I was their wife or because I gave birth to their child, and not just because I "belonged" to them.

"Was there anyone or anywhere you felt you belonged?" she asks.

I know the answer to her question instantly, but I don't respond right away. I let myself really feel it in my bones before I speak it.

"With my Old Man."

The Old Man—Summer 1995

I see him from where I stand at the edge of Granny's carport, rolling smoke lingering above his lips.

"Hey, Old Man, wanna go for a ride?" I holler.

It is a beautiful day—and a hot one at that. No better way to cool off than wind blowing through my curls. I long for a drive. Just a quick trip down to the boat dock at the end of the street to see how high the water is. The one where I learned to fish, skip rocks, and navigate the banks of Lake Cumberland with a raft and an old trolling motor we rigged up.

"Nope," he says. "Too much work to do around the house. Maybe 'morrow." His oversized Levi's barely cover his behind as he storms about the yard to look busier than he is. He often wore tracks in the grass from hours of pacing, reminding me of a chicken looking for seed. Between him and Poppy, the green blades take quite a beating.

The work is never done, he says.

Gotta keeps busy.

Idle hands are the devil's workshop.

His light blue cotton button-up stops just a couple of inches from his belly button. His graying chest hair stands up wildly, and his sweat stains are prominently displayed on the shirt, which he wears too much. His hair is disheveled, ombed to one side to hide the early emerging bald spot in the back. His eyes are a soft blue, and, aside from the color, they look a lot like mine.

Cigarette ashes dust his chest and look like glitter to a little girl vying for her daddy's attention. A smudge painted across his right cheek makes me wonder what he's been up to. Probably up and under that old truck again. The tiredness left in his eyes tells me he didn't sleep well or got up early when the rooster started to crow to make a fried egg and a burnt bologna sandwich with a slab of mayo.

My favorite.

I notice everything.

I drop my head as dramatically as I can, in a way much like Granny taught me, and sulk something awful. I feel his eyes looking over at me, but I refuse to look back.

"Get the keys. Meet me in five."

I snicker but turn my head so he can't see me. *I knew he'd change his mind.* He always does.

I skip off to grab the keyring, which he always leaves lying in the driver's seat. I rattle the cluster in my hand as loudly as possible, hoping he'll come on sooner than the five minutes he promised. I am just as antsy as he is, always wanting to be on the go—always needing my mind stimulated in some way.

I scooch over the bench seat to the truck's passenger side about the time he walks up to the window. Distracted by Granny and her purple pants waving something in her hand nearly one hundred feet in the distance, probably the ham salad sandwich, I don't notice him at first. I give her a good ole southern head nod.

I catch a whiff of smoke again. The Old Man, still watching me outside my window. I give the crank-turn handle about five good churns until I start to feel the burn of cigarette smoke seeping in.

"What the hell are ya doing?" he asks.

"Um, sittin' here," I say. "What's it look like?" *He sure does like to bicker.*

"You're on the wrong side, Littl'n. I ain't a driving."

"Well, then, who is?"

"You are."

"Dad." I look at him, cockeyed. "I'm nine. I can't drive. At least not legally."

"You ain't goin' to jail. And if you do, they'll bring ya right back," he says with a shit-eatin' grin growing across his face.

He is probably right.

He opens the door from the outside and nudges me over. I scoot past the cigarette burns in the cloth and pass what is left of the stain from the spilled orange soda he bought me last weekend until I am behind the wheel.

"Ugh. And it's a stick?" I say. "I can't drive a stick."

There's a long pause, but we never break eye contact. *I really do have his eyes, even if they aren't blue.*

"I guess today is the day you learn, Littl'n."

I open the driver's side door and hop out of the pickup truck in a frenzy. I look up and down the metal storage building behind the trailer where he keeps all his knickknacks and doodads for the upkeep of the property. High and low, throwing up anything that might stand in my way, searching for anything that might help me. He looks at me through the windshield with his eyebrow raised like I've gone mad.

"What the hell are you doing?" he asks for a second time with his head half stuck out the window.

"Lookin' for a helmet, Old Man," I say.

"A helmet? What do you need that for? We're driving a truck, not riding a motorcycle."

I don't answer. He already knows why I am looking for a helmet. And he already knows that I ain't gonna find one.

———

"So why *did* you need a helmet?" my therapist asks.

"I didn't *need* one. I just needed to *look* for one," I say.

"I'm not sure I follow."

It was something the Old Man and I did. Spoke to each other without saying anything—through gestures, mostly dramatic ones. I was telling him that I was afraid—that I *was* going to drive, not because he told me to, only because he told me I *could*.

"I wanted him to know I was afraid without telling him I was afraid," I say.

"Was this a normal form of communication for the two of you?"

It was. He understood my smart-aleck attitude, and he embraced it. It gave him a good laugh, made him think a little, and kept him on his toes.

"Yes," I say.

"Why couldn't you just tell him you were scared?"

"We didn't talk like that. We didn't express feelings. We didn't share our thoughts unless they came out in a fit of anger," I giggle.

"Well, how'd you learn to communicate with him that way?"

"Don't know. Just happened." I say.

"Did your siblings interact with your dad like this, too?"

I shake my head. "No—just me." He was close with my brother, probably because he was the only boy and the oldest, but they always fought. My dad said my brother was just like my Poppy, and my Poppy said my dad was just like my brother. Their communication involved arguments and an occasional fistfight, and that's about it. They never apologized or addressed the issue, just waited until they cooled off and acted like it never happened.

That didn't work for me.

I needed something different but didn't know what that was back then. I communicated in the way I was programmed to, nonverbally and sometimes with avoidance. I hadn't realized until now that this isn't healthy.

"What was it you needed back then?"

"Emotional safety—maybe a hug. I don't know," I say, struggling a bit with the honesty of it.

I couldn't remember being hugged by my mom. I couldn't remember being encouraged to share my feelings with my dad, which would have been too much for someone to process, so I kept them inside. I never had the opportunity to practice communication, problem-solving, and all the things necessary for a healthy relationship to grow.

"You know, I chose to date people that I thought needed fixing," I say. After hearing it aloud, I realize that was kind of an off-the-wall comment. But it fell out of my mouth as if it needed to be said.

"You were baking cookies instead of picking ones that were ready to eat."

"Cookies?" I ask.

"Yeah, baking cookies. You are trying to make people into what you think you need instead of seeing them for what they are, not just for what they could be," she says.

"Okay, I get it. I thought I was choosing people that needed fixing, but I was really the one that needed the help."

"I think you're right," she says. "That's a pretty common thing for people to do."

So that was it, that's what I am—a cookie baker. I'd been picking people who were still baking, taking a chance on what'd they be once they were done.

"It's often generational. We pass down unhealthy patterns to those who come after us without meaning to, and sometimes without realizing it," she says.

I think about Pop and Gran, how they were the only two in the family who stayed together, and I often wonder why. He was like that old grandfather clock that hung in the living room to me—predictable, which was comforting. I wondered if Granny felt the same. He'd say the same words each time he saw me, always in the same way, always with the same hands that wore a gold wedding band on the left and a Masonic ring on the right.

"You said you needed physical touch back then. What did it feel like to be hugged by your family?" she asks.

I think back to those times walking out the door to go back to Mom's, hearing Granny yell "love ya" right before she took a long sip of piping hot coffee. I didn't even feel comfortable enough to say it back. She must have told me hundreds of times without me saying a word. I thought about the occasional love pats and the lengths I would go to avoid them.

"Weird," I admit.

Poppy—Summer 1995

H ey there, Punkin-eater," Poppy says as I come in through the garage after the
drive with Dad. He reaches his hand out for me to rub my head against like
an old house cat might, and I do.

"Where'd ya go?" he says. "Out looking at houses again?"

As if he even has to ask. He knows it's my favorite thing to do. He tells me I
will be an architect when I grow up. The history, the rooflines, and the charm of
homes across Somerset, Kentucky, speak what feels like a secret language to me.
The older houses are found on College Street, the lake houses are on the south end
of town, and all the farms are to the north. What fun we have driving around,
comparing them all.

"Want a cold drink?" Granny asks from in front of the stove.

"Whatcha got?"

"Whatcha want?"

"I'll take a glass of moonshine," I tell her with a smile. She knows I am joking
but shakes her head and glares over at Poppy, giving him the side-eye. She knows
he's the one that told me about moonshine.

"You're too young for moonshine," Poppy pipes in. "Gotta be at least twelve
for that," he says with a raspy voice and a wink. All the while, he never skips a beat
in his game of solitaire.

I let loose a little chuckle, shake my head like Granny always does, and keep on walking through the dining room toward the bathroom. The hall is dark. The lights are turned off. I hear Pop's voice in my head: *No electricity is needed when the sun does a perfectly good job heatin' the place.*

If that penny-pincher of a man can save a nickel by working ten times as hard, he'll do it. He keeps his loose change in an old cigar box in his bedroom, and when it gets full, he takes it up to the bank on the town square and deposits it into his savings account. He likes to keep cash, though. He says it makes him feel sophisticated. He'll slip it in my rolled-up fist every now and then when he is feeling extra generous, then he'll tell me not to speak a word of it to Granny.

She knows where he keeps his money, too, and little does Pop know, she does the exact same thing—slips me a twenty and tells me not to tell him. This is the Mitchell way—always a *don't tell Gran, don't tell Mom, don't tell Pop, don't tell Dad*—everything's a secret, everything's a mystery.

Walking down that hallway, I am tempted to sneak back to the room and see how many quarters I can stuff in my pockets without them noticing, but I don't. Instead, I stop mid-stride, directly in front of the bathroom.

What has that crazy woman done now?

Something is different. The door handle still doesn't latch all the way, but that isn't it. There is a new maroon rug to match the cracked plastic toilet seat cover, but that's not it either.

Maybe it's wallpaper. *Did she hang wallpaper?*

My eyes move up the walls, curiously. Butterflies float across the ceiling—small ones, big ones, and yellow ones with black spots.

She didn't. Why on Earth would she?

I remind myself why I came into the bathroom in the first place. I need a bobby pin to keep the windblown hair out of my eyes. She keeps them in the same metal cup with tulip-shaped cutouts in the top drawer and has for as long as I can remember.

It is ninety degrees outside, and it feels about that in the house, too.

"Eugene, why's it so hot in here?" I yell from the hallway. I call him by his first name when I am being ornery. He acts like he doesn't like it, but I know he does.

"Hot? It ain't hot," he huffs under his breath.

"The thermostat says eighty-three degrees."

No response. I know he hears me, but he acts like he doesn't.

Her footsteps sound like a baby elephant getting closer and closer to me. Standing in the hall's shadow, Granny's hands are perched on her wide and fluffy hips. "Now, Kasey Renee, you know that old crazy man won't turn the air on until the first of June. That's the rule. That ain't 'til Sunday, so you'll just have to wait."

I mean, what do you say to that? It wouldn't matter what it was; he won't change his mind. He never does. What he says goes, and everyone knows it. He's the voice of reason, the deciding vote, the constant in the family—the only one you don't challenge, right in line before Mom.

I know better than to touch the thermostat even though I want to so badly, because I fear the consequences. Not so much for what he would do or say to me, but that he would assume my misbehavior was Gran's fault. To him, this was no different than touching the television remote during *Wheel of Fortune* or turning on a light after nine at night. You just don't do it.

I walk back into the bathroom, toes curled up in the shag toilet rug, and go on about my business. I wet my hair with water as cold as possible, slick it back with a comb, and plug a bobby pin under the band to hold all the stray hairs down. Then I go back out to the living room, eager to see who won the game of solitaire.

"Hey, Pop. You win?"

He pushes the crystal bowl filled to the brim with fresh boiled peanuts over in my direction. I scoop up a handful, blow off the heat with one big puff, and plop them in my mouth, wiping the leftover salt onto my little tan legs.

"I always win," he says with a wink.

"Did you see what Granny did to the bathroom?"

He shakes his head incessantly, rubs his mustache, and avoids eye contact. He saw it. I know he did.

"I don't go in Granny's bathroom. If she wants to carry on like a garden fairy, she can as long as I don't have to know about it," he says. "Shew! Butterflies in a bathroom make about as much sense as tits on a bull."

He gives a husky chuckle, and just when I thought I'd slip by him, he snakes a wiry arm out to wrap around my waist to pull me close for a quick instant, fitting me in tight against his chest and collarbone. The squeeze is fast, just long enough for me to breathe in the scent of his Ivory soap, which just so happens to be covering the smell of sweat, the secret draws of cigarettes, *and* the starch Granny uses to make his shirts stand up.

Then he lets me go, my feet falling gently onto the tile floor.

Okay then. They've had it out over the butterflies, so I don't say another word. I know when to shut my mouth, and this is one of those times.

Poppy likes it that we think alike. It's as if he's trying to pass the ornery gene down to me; it connects us, much like the helmet and the Old Man, and Granny in the garden. I give them each a second glance, wondering how they act when I'm not around—who's the first to apologize, who's the first to say "I love you," and who works the hardest to keep the relationship going. After all, this was the only model I had in my life for what a marriage looks like.

"Well, ya two lovebirds, I'm outta here. I'll see ya back on Sunday."

"How did you view your grandparents' relationship?" my therapist asks.

I hadn't thought much of it, but I guess I always saw them as a duo. Like Tom and Jerry, Lucy and Ethel, or Fred and Barney. When I thought of Granny, I thought of Poppy and vice versa—never one without the other.

"I thought of them as fine."

I mean, yes, there was bickering, but that's how they showed love to one another. I'm sure they didn't always agree, but at the end of the day, they each lay in the bed in the back bedroom, pulled up the covers, and said, "See ya in the morning." I never knew one of them to spend a night without the other. I never saw them having arguments where one leaves, even though Mom said it used to happen. Perhaps Pop did that earlier in their marriage but grew out of it by the time I came around. I never heard either one say, "I'm done." They were always where they were supposed to be—at home. They were my constant, my predictable; they were my escape.

"They were the only love that I ever saw that worked."

"And by *worked*, do you mean didn't end in divorce?" she asks.

That is a good question. I guess that is what I mean. I nod my head.

"How did they react when you and Frank split up?"

"I don't know. They never said a word about it," I say.

"How did you feel when the three of you were together?"

"Important."

I knew if I made Granny mad, which I did often, I could come back the next day, and it would be like nothing ever happened. I felt like she loved me unconditionally. No grudges. No contingencies. Just love like a grandmother is supposed to love a granddaughter. I felt like that until I became an adult. Then she judged me. Maybe it was just her age, or the fact that she was so set in her ways, but our relationship changed the older I got.

"Is that how you see yourself when you're a grandma?"

Partially, yes. I mean, yes, to the unconditional love part, not so much to the relationship with Pop. He was the head of the household and the voice that she looked to for final decisions. I never understood or agreed with that, even though she told me that's the way the Bible said it should be. I don't know why they stayed together—if they settled, if it was because of my dad, or if they figured they were too old to split up. Maybe they really did love one another, or had a mutual respect, I'm not sure. Even with his old-fashioned "man of the household" role, Poppy still seemed to respect Granny, but I don't know the true answer to any of those questions—I never got the chance to ask.

Once I became an adult, they didn't understand me, and, instead of trying, they pushed away all that was unfamiliar. They were set in their ways, and I was just coming into my own. I dated people they didn't think I should date. They were raised to believe that white girls should only date white boys. I moved away even though they thought I should be happy where I was. I had a baby when I wasn't married. There were so many things of which they disapproved. There were so many things that pushed us apart.

"The only people I ever felt accepted me started to reject me, too," I say.

I quietly say this multiple times inside my head each time my heart starts to ache. Each time I start to feel a loss, I make excuses for them.

They did the best they could.

They did what they knew.

It's how they were raised.

Each time I want a Mr. Pibb and a Little Debbie, I remind myself why I can't just drop in like I used to. I battle with myself over them often. Maybe it is because I haven't forgiven them, or maybe I don't understand why I battle myself over them, and why they couldn't accept me and love me unconditionally.

My therapist interrupts my thinking: "What did that little nine-year-old girl need from her family, Kasey?" Then she adds, "Tell me more about your childhood."

I do what most clients do when their therapist asks an important question they don't want to answer. I lie.

"It was great."

She knows there is more. Her raised brow tells me so. "Did you experience anything traumatic as a kid?"

The only thing that comes to mind was when I was bit by a dog, but I force myself to think deeper. Everyone has trauma; whether it's a big one or a little one, there's trauma within us all.

"I'm sorry, but I'm trying to think. There's nothing major that comes to mind."

"You've described spending a lot of time with your grandparents," she says.

I was at their house every chance I got. I liked it there because of the endless amounts of snacks, and I could have a soda anytime I wanted one. I could be as independent as I wanted to be. I could dream as loud as I wanted and that was okay. I was free. There was no such thing as noise to Granny.

"What was it like at your mom's?"

Different.

It was completely different at her house. I always wanted to be somewhere else, not to get away from her, but because I liked to stay busy, and she liked to sleep.

"Where was your mother when you were there?"

"Her bedroom, mostly."

"Where were you?"

"Outside, mostly."

We lived in an apartment complex, and there were quite a few kids around that I could play with—that I could get into trouble with. That's where I crashed through someone's sliding glass door on a banana bike. It's where my attempt at riding the break in the concrete landed me a nice clean slash across my left wrist. That scar gives any nurse attempting to put in an IV enough reason to screen for suicidal thoughts. It's where the other kids and I nearly got banned from the neighborhood for chopping down a tree. I can't even tell you why we did it.

I did anything, and everything, to give my mom space—anything to make the days pass until I could go back to Granny and Poppy's.

I lived outside in the creek that ran in front of my apartment, riding my bike or building forts up in the "secret" part of the woods surrounding the property.

"She lived inside, struggling emotionally, until she met my stepdad. That was the first time I saw her come back to life."

"If that was the case, then what was she to you before him?"

Gone.

"Is this how you felt as a child—the first nine years of your life—like your mom was gone?" she asks.

I don't know. I don't remember anything with her before nine. She met my stepdad shortly after that, I think. What must it have felt like to have an emotionally absent mother, even if it wasn't her fault? Even if she was doing the best she could.

"Have you ever talked to her about it?" she asks.

"No."

The thought of talking to my mom, or anyone in my family, about my feelings makes my stomach ache. She'd be defensive. She'd take it as a personal attack against her when that's not my intention.

"Do you think I should?"

I ask the question, but I don't really want to know the answer. She nods her head, and that makes me nervous. I am committed to therapy and to this process, so if my therapist tells me to do something, I'll do it, but that doesn't mean I want to. I want to improve my relationship with my mom, get closer to her, and make sure she knows that I'm always here for her, but I don't know how. I don't know where to start.

Caring for your mental health wasn't as accepted back when I was a kid like it is today. You were judged when you were honest about your needs and asked for help. She told me about a time she asked once, told my Granny and Poppy that she was severely depressed, and it was used against her. My mom is a very proud woman. I know she wouldn't have wanted to feel judged. From that time on, I bet she suffered in silence for that reason. It's what you were expected to do—what women were expected to do.

I pause for a moment just to breathe. It hurts to imagine a world where you can't be honest with yourself or anyone else out of fear that you'd be condemned. That your depression is a sign of being "crazy." That your mood swings are a side effect of being a woman. That the very thing that makes you human also makes you feel alone and dehumanized. It's hard to imagine a world where I couldn't do what I'm doing right now, getting help.

I release the air from my lungs, slowly. "What else are you going to ask me to do?"

"What do you think you need to do?"

She's really putting this back on me, isn't she? Now I know how my clients must have felt when I said things like this to them.

Confused—November 2021

Dear Journal,

Remembering, even something as simple as who my family was to me when I was a child, has been hard. I blocked out more things than I ever realized. I spent hours crying about what played out in my adult life within my family that I nearly forgot what they were like when I was a kid.

I can remember them and some of the stories of us together. Like how my sister and her ex-husband took me bowling with their church friends on Wednesday nights. I remember my brother taking me to the grocery store when I was tiny, getting a kick out of telling me to holler at people from the car window. I remember times with Poppy and Granny, of course. But I remember only a few stories about me and my mom.

When I think about her, I find my body resisting the memories of my Inner Child. I don't know what I was like with her. Did Mom somehow suppress my Inner Child? Was my Inner Child afraid to be herself around my mother? Was she confused by her? Why can't I remember?

~Confused

For You (#Remember)

Dear Seeker,

Going back in time, thinking about the child you once were, can feel scary. It was for me. It can also be sad. There's a lot of negativity that comes along with dredging up the past, which is why you hear people say, *Don't look back. You can't change the past. Focus on the future.* And they're partially right. You can't change the past, but you can change the way you think about it and the meaning you make of it. And that, my friend, is powerful.

A former consulting client of mine and trauma specialist, Rachel Harrison, once told me that our memories are like grapes—little networks connected on a vine. When we activate one, we find more, and more. When you allow yourself to Remember and let go of the resistance you feel, you gain so much more access to hidden, blocked, or repressed memories.

Those emotions can bring about all sorts of new experiences, like how you view yourself in different phases of your life: baby, child, teen, and adult. The person you were as a child never goes away because you grow older. That little girl doesn't just grow up and cease to be. She doesn't just become a woman and leave her younger self behind. That little girl still lives inside of you, and she always will. Part of your subconscious, she's called your Inner Child. She was picking up messages since you were in utero, before you could ever process life physically and emotionally. She holds emotions, memories, and beliefs from the past and hopes and dreams for the future.

And to find joy again, you must first find *her*. Then you must learn to love her.

That's what we're doing here, we're *remembering* so that we can find *her* again. Looking this far back can be upsetting. I want you to be able to review your past from a grounded and balanced place. Snuggle up with your favorite blanket, grab your smoothest writing pen, and put on some music that helps you feel safe. Then use these questions as a starting point to write in your notebook, but allow yourself the freedom to create your own experience. Don't limit yourself to these instructions.

What is your first childhood memory?

Who were the people who made the biggest impact on you emotionally?

What feelings did you attach to each person in your life?

What is your first memory of feeling safe?

What was your first memory of feeling emotionally supported?

Who made you feel safe and how?

Who did you turn to when you needed something?

Who made you feel free?

What is your favorite childhood memory?

What inspired you? Scared you?

What did you do when you were afraid?

How did your family show love? Anger? Joy? Fear?

Who was allowed or expected to show these feelings and who wasn't?

What did you long for as a child?

How can you start having compassion for that little girl?

Your Inner Child can guide you toward answers you may have in your life right now—maybe she can move you closer to what you've been searching for. Maybe your tendencies toward unhealthy relationships, seeking love and belonging, and chasing success are manifestations of an unmet need of hers? Maybe it has been your adult self, trying to meet the needs that she went an entire childhood without. You could have been searching, without even knowing, to fill a void or heal an old wound.

Your Inner Child may be little; she may be buried deep inside of you, but she's powerful. She's influential—critical to who you are and how you feel right now. She directs the path you take in your search toward fulfillment. She can tell you so much about yourself and how you got where you are right now, so how about you listen to her?

Take cues from your body and challenge your mind to do things that might feel hard or scary. But also have compassion for yourself and don't rush the process just to check it off the list so you can finish the book. I know you overachieving types are already giving yourself a deadline! It's okay to keep reading, even if you're not actively participating in each part.

You are on a journey, one with me as your guide, but ultimately *you* are in control.

Now, how would you describe that little girl who lives inside of you? Answer that question in your notebook, along with these (remember, they're just a springboard for unfathomable other questions inside you):

What does she dream of?

What lights her up?

What does she still need?

Who does she need it from?

After you spend some time Remembering, it's important to know that you must let go of all the *buts* and *what-abouts*. Your needs aren't dependent on your feelings, crossing every item off your to-do list, making a certain salary, or ensuring every child has every privileged "thing" you tell yourself they need. It isn't performance based. It can't be earned. Your worth and having your needs met emotionally is intrinsic to you as a person. You may not feel it, but you deserve everything. Give that little girl a hug or hold her hand. While you both might not feel like you deserve it, you do. Tell her you will be with her on this journey and that she never has to worry about being alone again.

Your Back Porch Bestie,

K

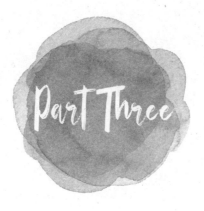

Part Three

Awareness
THE BIG THINGS

• Big Things are like fence posts
that shape our lives. •

"Trauma is not only the occurrence of events
and experiences, but the absence of love,
safety, trust, belonging, and connection."
~unknown

When we work toward more awareness in our lives, Big Things come to mind first; these are the moments that changed us. They can trick us into believing that we are defined by them, but that doesn't have to be true. Big Things are merely fence posts that help shape our lives. By gaining awareness of how they molded us, we can learn to use them in our quest for joy.

The Timeline—October 2021

As I gain more awareness of the feelings I have now and the messages I received as a child, I also notice that I need even more for positive change to occur.

There's been a shift since reintroducing myself to my Inner Child in those first few sessions of therapy. Since I told my therapist the stories of my Poppy, Granny, Mom, and the Old Man, I thought even more about the impact they had on me. It was like they came to life again in my heart.

Sometimes they feel like more than memories, and there are moments when I realize how much space they hold in my heart. Each are part of the Big Things that happened in my young life; yet somehow, up until now, I glossed over them like they weren't much of anything. My brain blocked some because what I don't remember can't hurt me. Right?

Or can it?

I know I need to make space to feel the bigness of those memories. That's the only way I'll understand why I keep putting myself back into relationships that are unhealthy. I need to understand why I'm triggered by a suitcase being packed or someone threatening to leave—or why I try to beat them to the punch. I need to figure out why I keep settling for unbaked cookies. I need to understand why noise bothers me when I loved it as a little girl. I need to figure out why joy doesn't exist, no matter how successful I have become.

To do all this, I need to lay out all the Big Things bare and become aware of how they shaped the direction my life took.

I love this fireplace.

That green tile must be original.

Wonder what kind of wood that is.

It reminds me of a tiger.

I'm so glad I put all these pictures up.

That one of Granny and the Old Man at the Wolf Creek Dam looks cool.

Do I have ADHD?

My office is cozy, just like I always wanted. It reminds me of Poppy's house and Granny's memory wall that I used to tease her about—a cluttered collage of photo frames showcasing everyone, even the third, fourth, and fifth cousins. The ledge is covered with gifts my consulting clients send me. Mostly stacks of books because they know what I like, but there are other things, too. A picture frame that my CFO, Jackie, made that says, "I love Taylor Swift." A fiddle from the 1700s. It was my Poppy's, or so my Old Man says. He took care of it through several generations, and my dad gave it to me a few weeks ago. And of course, all the photos pinned to the corkboard in my peripheral remind me of the past.

My favorite thing sits underneath the desk that holds all my Moleskine notebooks—a stuffed fox that's seen better days. My dad shot her on accident with a BB gun when he was just a boy. Granny walked deep into the trees at the Wolf Creek Dam looking for that fox because you weren't supposed to shoot the wildlife, but Dad didn't have much of a tendency to follow the rules. When she found it, she named it Foxy (creative, I know) and carried it, six shades of dead, back to the house. Tucked up under the food in the deep freeze to hide from Pop, it sat while she found someone to stuff it. Two months later, Foxy became a permanent fixture in the Mitchell family, complete with a diamond collar around her neck. She sat beside Granny's recliner in her living room until I asked the Old Man if I could have her. Now, she sits with me and scares every unsuspecting newbie who walks into my office.

Looking around at all the stuff I originally put up for inspiration, I realize courage is what I really need to continue in this process, because I'm scared, and I'm already resisting the work. Flooded with emotions, I feel immense loss. I miss being a kid at Granny and Poppy's—where they did everything for me, where I didn't have a care in the world. I miss the rides with the Old Man. I miss the fishing trips, roasting marshmallows, and setting out on a good long moped ride for the day. I miss sitting up in that maple tree, checking on how the garden was coming along, how the minnows we used for fishing bait looked like they were kissing. I miss the way I looked forward to what each day would bring.

I had so much joy back then; despite the hard times—despite my parents' divorce, the loneliness, all those things—I still felt it. *I need to know when I lost it,* where it went, and why it left me.

Once I allow myself to remember the people, the feelings, my Inner Child, everything else in my heart starts to open just like the vine of grapes that Rachel told me about. I tell my body to move, and my hands shuffle through the notebooks sitting above Foxy, until they find one with a few blank pages.

I discard a few notebooks as "too nice" for doodles, another couple as too small for the thoughts I'm trying to think. The one I settle on is larger than your average journal. A full 8½ by 11 inches and bright blue—big enough to think any thought I want. Big enough to draw out my entire life, all the events that stand out to me, significant or not. I need to get it out of my head and onto something tangible, just like Poppy and my Old Man used to do every morning under the big tree between their homesteads—they drew out the day.

Could I draw out my life?

Instead of planning what's coming, could I list what's been? Would that help me see something new? Instead of planning for my future like everyone says to do, what if I look back? What if I do the thing that no one wants to do? Lean into the resistance and go from there.

I settle in on the couch opposite those green wingbacks I love, prop my feet up against the coffee table like I did as a teen on the dash of Dad's truck, and poise my pen as if I'm going to write the most amazing sentence in the history of the world.

Instead I write, "Kasey's Timeline."

My head fills with whispers—*Should I start with "was born"? I don't even remember anything from when I was little. What is this going to prove anyway? I'm only dredging up things that make me sad or things that make me mad. This is not the mindset I need if I talk with my mom. Which, by the way, I'm definitely not doing.*

But, as if by magic, my body carries on while my brain chatters, as if it knows what the heart needs. I watch as words, dates, and feelings coincide with each appearance, and the whispers stop. I start at my first significant adult memory and fill in as much as I can until I get to the present. It takes hours, or longer, I don't know.

I look up from the page, only to see darkness peering in from the window. I have nowhere to be—no one waiting for me at home, so it doesn't really matter. I write more until my life, the good, the bad, the ugly, is laid out before me like a map, starting with the Big Things. It's nothing fancy, nothing I ever plan to show to anyone. It is just for me.

As I study the sequence of events, things start to click. Emotions that I pushed down are still there, just waiting to bring me back. Events, ones at the time I thought were random, were very connected, and I can see it now. Decisions that I thought were based on gut instincts were reactions to events and emotions I had repressed.

It's both enlightening and overwhelming. My stomach churns, and the tension in my upper back between my shoulder blades pulsates. There's so much about myself that I have never had the awareness to see.

I go back through the timeline, drawing out patterns and noticing themes. My Poppy would be proud of how I pick out the signs of a bigger picture. I notate upsetting and traumatic events with "t." I mark the moments I felt joy with a capital "J." As my finishing touch, I notate all the places I felt fear with a big black "F."

I don't like thinking of myself as a fearful person, but as I look through my life on paper, I can see a lot more fear and a lot less joy.

Frank—2002 to 2009

We meet during my junior year of high school. Frank is a year older than me. We date on and off through college until he drops out against his parents' wishes to start a business, and I run off to Chicago to find myself. When life doesn't work out as I imagine, I move back to my hometown, rent a bug-infested basement apartment for two hundred dollars a month, and give college another go. I resign myself to a normal, predictable, expected life like all the other good southern girls.

At twenty-two years old, I am too young to be a part of anything serious, but calling someone my husband feels grown-up and respectable—and that's what I think I want.

Turns out I don't know what I want.

Frank is athletic, well liked, and the life of the party. I am an introvert and don't have a lot of friends. He comes from a good family, with parents who are still married and seem happy. My family life is tumultuous, and my divorced parents have nothing nice to say about each other. He has grown up going on family vacations and eating sit-down dinners at restaurants that require reservations. I have never been on vacation, and Wendy's is the nicest place I've ever eaten. He has everything I don't.

When he asks me to marry him, of course, I say yes. Even if it isn't an actual proposal, and even if I find the ring wrapped up in a wad of toilet paper in his pocket one evening while we ride his street bike. To me, it is enough, even though there is no down-on-one-knee, no photographer to capture the moment, and no butterflies in my belly—it is enough.

I can see a life with him. We'll have a lovely brick house in the city, a couple of dogs, and maybe more one day. He'll work, and I'll teach and maybe even own a clothing boutique on the side. We'll have family dinners and go camping. That's what I see when I look at Frank—an opportunity for a nice, normal, happy life.

He'll spend each fall coaching little league football, and I'll sit on the sidelines wearing my team sweatshirt. We'll have a nice clawfoot bathtub and save up for Christmas all year. We'll go on vacation every summer and have a beautiful spring wedding near the water. I'll go dress shopping with a group of my closest girlfriends, toast champagne, and take a selfie when I find the perfect one. My dad will walk me down the aisle, and my mom will give me something borrowed and blue. They'll tell me they love me and want the best life for me. And for Frank.

No one tells me we aren't right for each other. No one says he is not the one—no one tells me I'm not ready. There is no heart-to-heart over hot chocolate with my mom to tell me how hard marriage will be and that *I* might not know enough about myself yet to know how to navigate a future with someone else. All I know is that he is the image of what I think a husband should look like, and I want to feel like I belong somewhere, even if it was to someone. It is about safety and finding a place for me; I think he just wants a wife.

I want someone to make me feel something.

We go together like oil and water, like fire and gasoline; the harder we fight to stay together, the deeper the wedge we create. I search outward for connection, meaning, and fulfillment, which causes jealousy, resentment, and unhealthy attachments. He pays the bills, sets up our accounts, and gives me money when I want to buy something. He calls the cable company when there is a problem, upgrades our cell phones, and purchases our vehicles. Back then, this is love, this is what men do in relationships, and it is the only kind I want because it is all I know exists.

He does the best he can for me financially—the way he was raised to care for a woman—but we bring out the worst in each other emotionally. He is super jealous, and I can't navigate a conflict to save my life. We spend most of our time arguing and have very little in common other than the fact that neither one of us knows when to cut bait and run.

When he looks at me, it doesn't feel the way I'd always imagined it is supposed to when you're in love. I don't feel a deep sense of connection and peace, and he knows something is missing, too. Throughout our relationship, he grasps at ways to satisfy me, but the harder he tries, the more I detach.

Something inside of me says no.

I want more, and so does he, even though he never tells me that. He doesn't ask me about my thoughts, feelings, or dreams; looking back now, I needed that. I need someone to make me feel like I matter in that way, too—I need a deep and meaningful connection. I need someone to grow alongside me and support me. I need a best friend.

We don't sleep in the same bed, and I tell myself it is because he snores. We don't hold hands when we walk down the street or into a restaurant. We don't cuddle on the couch watching a movie or get caught up in the moment when we lock eyes over breakfast. Our life is regimented, logical, and predictable—just like what I think I want. But it is missing something—*I* am missing something, and that is something Frank has no control over.

There are good times at the beginning and bad times in the end. When our relationship takes a downward spiral, he points out my insecurities to remind me that I am flawed in every way imaginable. He isn't stupid, and he knows how to hurt me. Over time, I learn how to hurt him back. Every time I move closer to finding my true self, he senses it and reacts. It is a constant charade of give and take.

After a year of threatening divorce, with no real change happening, I do whatever the hell I want to. I am just as much the problem in our relationship as he is, if not more, but Frank doesn't want to give up on me easily. We are both too young and stubborn to quit. It takes more than six years to cut our losses. Years of hurting each other and everyone else around us until it finally blows up in my face. And just like that, in what seemed like a moment, it is done. Over.

He stands upstairs in the media room of our 1920 Tutor, on shag carpet, while I sit with my head in my hands on the sectional.

"Go!" he says. "Go do whatever the hell you want. Go find yourself. Go chase your dreams. Go be with someone else; you know you want to. You've always wanted more. You can't settle down. Go be with that guy from my cousin's wedding reception; I saw how he looked at you—how you looked at him."

Who is he talking about?

"Who, Victor?"

He doesn't respond.

Why is he bringing up Victor?

I don't hear anything Frank says after that. My thoughts are somewhere else altogether—somewhere new, interesting, somewhere that challenges me. *He told me to go. This is my out.* My mind leaves that conversation and that relationship, and it moves on to something that begs to ask the question, "What if there is more out there for me?"

My identity has been wrapped up in being Frank's for quite some time. I am too young to know who I was before Frank. I certainly don't know who I am *with* Frank, and I really don't know who I am *after* Frank. I just know that Frank is not good for me, and I am not good for Frank.

I can't speak for him, but if I had to guess, I'd say he would agree that our relationship was over for a long time before the conversation that day, and it is a good thing that we are finally making it official. It is my first big watershed moment—the moment that forces a change. A culmination of the lessons I'd learned is in my hands, and it is up to me as to what to do with it.

At twenty-five years old, I am faced with a loss, and with that loss comes a choice. I can go out into the world, chase down my dreams, bounce from place to place, sights set on anything or anyone who makes me feel something . . . Or I can turn the other way. I can look within, inside myself for truth, for meaning, for what it is that I truly want out of life.

Motherhood–2009

A month later, in February, I sign up for an adult ballet class. I need a distraction from a life that is now drastically different from the normal one I imagined. Frank had always been my constant, and now he is gone.

I tell myself I am there to work on myself, strengthen my core—you know, all the things that twenty-five-year-olds need to do. Mostly I need *not* to think about how messed up my life is.

I show up with a friend, stretch out on the floor in a circle of other tentatively friendly women, and instantly feel sick—sick enough to stop at Walgreens on the way home to grab a bottle of Pepto and a pregnancy test.

It is positive.

―――――――

Everyone tells me not to eat a big meal before I go into labor. No one warns me that no matter how much you prepare, childbirth is about as unpredictable as a game of roulette.

I crave Mexican in early September 2009, so I stop at my favorite place after work. I still have another five weeks before I am due, and I have three dogs to walk before bed. A chimichanga, rice, and beans down, and a bowl of queso to top it off, I feel good. I don't mind eating alone; in fact, I kind of like it. It gives me time to reflect and relax. I get my check, pay it, and drive the short distance home.

Three tangled leashes pull me zigzag down the old downtown street. My dogs' little white tails wag as if they've been waiting for this moment all day. I'm ready for a good night's sleep, so I walk them a little farther than I typically do, pushing myself a little harder than normal.

When the four of us barely have the strength to lift our legs, we head back home. I pull off the shoes from my swollen feet and raise them up on the ottoman in the corner of the nursery. I've done a lot of work to it in the last seven and a half months, and even though I don't have much money, it has come together well. I take a few breaths, sink down into the glider, and feel a tightness in my stomach.

Contractions.

It's normal at this stage in the pregnancy, right? I pay close attention because of the pre-term pregnancy complications I've already experienced. Over the next hour, they are down to three minutes apart and regular. I am restless and suffering from a headache. The pharmacy is right down the street, so I think it is best to grab some Tylenol before it gets too late.

By the time I pull into the parking lot, the contractions are harder and stronger.

Maybe I should just swing by labor and delivery and let my doctor check me.

I don't want to burden anyone, but I don't want to give birth at home either, so I decide to stop.

"You're being admitted," the nurse checking my vitals tells me. "You're dilated and the baby's heart rate is up."

I wait until I can't stand the pain any longer, then I call my mom.

"Head this way," I say. "You're about to be a grandma."

It feels like the longest birth ever, but it is the only one I've ever had, so I can't be certain. My doctor, a tall, thin woman about my sister's age, tries to convince me to have a Cesarean section. She tells me it will be faster, but I say no.

When Maime is finally born and I can hold her, I struggle to find the words to express how I feel. The tension in my chest and the fuzziness in my head are things I've never experienced. I am excited, scared, sad, and about twenty other feelings all at the same time.

In my head I say to her, "I'm your mommy," but that sounds too strange to say out loud, so I keep it hidden. The more time I spend with her, the more comfortable I become. I stare at her, take pictures of her, and imagine all the ways my life is about to change.

It's the night before I'm scheduled to go home, and I sit up in the bed, feeding her. She is so hungry and loves to be held. Her eyes are dark blue, the color of most babies' eyes, but they are already starting to focus. At first they zero in on the nightgown that I am wearing. Then I watch them move to other things. It makes me nervous that she is so close to me, in such an intimate way.

I keep watching her, ignoring the glitches in the flourescent lighting up above and the sounds of other babies crying from down the hall. And then, it is as if our surroundings fall away, and all I see is her. My baby.

As quietly as I can, and with an unnatural force, I whisper, "I love you, Maime Adeline. I. Love. You."

Because I believe that even if it feels strange, it needs to be said. She deserves that.

Eggs–2013

I am twenty-nine; Maime is four; and Poppy is sick.

He refuses to eat, and he's lost his spunk. I am the only one who can make him drink the chocolate Ensure the doctors continue to give him, but he fights me tooth and nail every time. "It tastes like metal," he says. "I ain't hungry," he argues.

There is not a diagnosis that has given us any answers or peace of mind since he's been sick.

I am the primary point of contact for his discharging physician aside from Granny. Still, they prefer to talk to me because I come across as the most clear-headed one in the family. They think Granny is senile, and rightfully so, because she spent Pop's stint in the hospital raising hell about the nurse whom she accused of flirting with her husband.

My phone rings.

"This is Kasey."

"Hello, this is Dr. Tate. I want to let you know that your grandfather is being discharged today."

"Are you sure that's a good idea?" I ask.

I am by his side when the doctor calls. Pop perks up and begs to go home. He looks me dead in the face and says, "I want to go home, Kasey." He never calls me by my name. I am his Punkin, and I am not sure I like the sound of anything else coming from his mouth.

I don't know if he means *home*-home, the one on Slate Branch, or the heavenly home I overheard him talk about with the deacons at church when I was a kid, but either way, I don't want him to go. If he goes back to Slate Branch Road, he'll die there. If he stays here in the hospital, eventually, he'll die here, too. He wants to be home, and I respect that, but home will never be the same without him.

The doctors are adamant that it is time to go, so we go. We order a hospital bed that is to be delivered to the house by the time we get there. It is too large to fit in the bedroom, so they set it up in the living room instead. I tell them to prop it up right in front of the television, which is conveniently programmed for his favorite shows, even though he barely has the strength to watch them.

We make the short trip back to the house and get him situated exactly like I imagined. I take a seat on the couch beside his hospital bed in the living room and think about what home means to him—about what home means to me.

"Gran, how 'bout some scrambled eggs?" he says.

"You can't eat eggs, Poppy. The doctor said NO solid food."

I can see he's tired, and the toll that all the moving around has taken has been great.

"I'll be back in the morning, Pop. Give Granny hell while I'm gone," I say with a smile. He doesn't smile back. I touch his hand and the ridges in his not-so-manicured fingernails, and pat down his disheveled hair just like he used to do to me.

I look at him for what feels like the last time, taking everything in—his weak eyes and distant mind—and my heavy heart is already somewhere far beyond where I could have ever imagined it would be. I watch Granny walk into the kitchen ahead of me to rummage through the refrigerator. I follow close behind her.

"Take care of him, Gran, but don't feed him eggs," I say as I walk out the garage door.

On the way back to my little rental house on Richardson Drive, the two-bedroom with a basement infested with black mold that I could barely afford, I stay quiet. No radio. No music. No nothing.

I turn it all off.

I turn off the music again.

It is just me and the road, in bone-chilling silence, mourning the death of a man who is physically still here, mourning a life that I know I will soon no longer have, mourning the only place that has ever been my home.

———

I get there before the ambulance does the following morning. I stuff my hands down in the pocket of the Chicago School of Medicine hoodie that I stole from my friend's condo. I tell myself to be strong. Be brave. Don't cry. It takes everything I have to walk back into that living room, the one with all the memories—the Christmas mornings, the evening TV watching, the company visiting. I know I should have never left him there. But I did, and I must see him again—even if it is one last time, even if I know that's not how I want to remember him.

I look up to see the grandfather clock mounted to the paneled wall, the one that has been there my entire life, but I can't read the time.

He is already gone.

He is home.

I am anywhere but.

A plate of half-eaten scrambled eggs sits by his bedside.

Everything happens quickly. The arrangements, taking care of Granny, and dropping Maime off with Frank so she doesn't have to go through a funeral at her age. But I forget to check myself.

"Poppy's funeral will be in two days. Eleven o'clock in the morning," Dad says.

I am weak, weaker than I am comfortable feeling. At first, I think that it's just the stress catching up with me. All these emotions must go somewhere, after all. But then I feel something different—something within my body. When I check, I see blood. Then more blood. Enough that it scares me. I call my "female doctor," as my dad likes to call it, and she tells me to come in right away.

"You're hemorrhaging," she says. "You need a D and C right now."

"A what?" I ask, already half in a panic. "Why?"

"You're pregnant. I will need to do an ultrasound; then I'm admitting you to the hospital for surgery."

The ultrasound shows an amniotic sac that is abnormal in shape, and that is all.

"Nothing developed in the sac," the doctor explains. "And at this point, nothing ever will. But if you don't have surgery, you will bleed out and you could die."

It is less than twelve hours until Poppy's funeral.

I don't tell anyone; I am too ashamed. Because of company policy, something about liabilities and risk, the ambulance transports me from the doctor's office to the ER. I am given a plastic bracelet, asked if I know what procedure I am about to receive, and left alone in a makeshift room to wait on a nurse to wheel me back for anesthesia. I am told that I am the first on the list for surgery.

At 8 AM, two hours after arriving, I am awake.

"When can I leave?" I ask.

I know they need to observe me to ensure there are no complications, but I don't know how long that takes.

An hour passes, and by 9 AM they tell me they are preparing my discharge paperwork. The nurse wants to know who is driving me home.

"My boyfriend."

I lie. I don't have anyone to drive me home. I don't have anyone at all.

Frank and I are over for good, and all I want is to feel loved again. I thought I found "the One" in an ER physician I met while I was completing practicum hours for a college program at a nearby hospital. But one night while working together on a patient with a broken arm, he bent over to pick up the casting mold that fell onto the floor, and a wedding band fell from the pocket in his scrubs. He is married and had been lying to me our entire relationship—even showing me divorce papers that were apparently fake (you can buy these online now, apparently).

I've dodged a bullet with him. After all, he is the reason I am here having surgery right now, and he's nowhere to be found.

After I sign the orders and take the prescription medication the nurse hands me for pain, I sneak off toward the parking lot where I originally left my car for my office visit, hoping no one will notice. Luckily, the hospital is just in a different building on the campus of the medical complex, but the parking lot is the same. I have an hour-long drive home, and I must change clothes before I get to the funeral home.

I am lonely.

I've lost Frank. I've lost the beginning of a baby. I've lost our patriarch, the only man who can keep my family together.

It feels like I have lost myself, too.

It is a death, which happens every day. We lose loved ones, and there's nothing we can do to change it, but this feels like more than that. A man who was always so strong and stoic, who was each person's rescuer, is lying empty in a casket lined with silk and covered in white roses. There is nothing he can do for any of us now; he can't even hold the glasses up on the bridge of his nose. He lies there so helpless, so innocent, but so incredibly gone.

Blame–August 2013

Pop's passing does exactly what I thought it would do. It changes us all.

⎯⎯⎯⎯

The most pleasant memories of my childhood are at his home. I never realized how comforted I felt by the traditions that happened there. That gave me enough grounding to feel like I still had a family, even when I was a young adult out on my own, trying to make a life for myself.

Thanksgiving dinner. Granny was a helluva cook, and this was my favorite meal of the year. The country ham, roasted turkey, mashed potatoes made from scratch, dressing that I'd love to remember how to make—the homemade pumpkin pie with a dollop of chilled Cool Whip, pecan pie with a Granny-fied design on top. The smells of that house when I walked through the door were always comforting and familiar.

"Hope ya came hungry," Granny said from behind a cast iron skillet with lard popping.

"You know I'll never turn down a good meal, Gran."

Christmas morning. The way Poppy sat eagerly perched in his recliner in the far-right corner of the living room, holding a trash bag big enough to stuff all of us grandkids in it, still makes me giggle. Not a shred of paper could make its way to the carpet without him scurrying over to pick it up. Paying no mind to us sprawled out in our Christmas pajamas, reaching for the gifts like they were hotcakes. He never noticed the Teddy Ruxpin that was the hottest gift one year or the baby dolls that piled up. He focused on one thing: keeping his floor clean.

Nightly supper. This was a thing growing up. Every evening, right about the time the men come home from work, a hot meal is served. Granny doesn't cook supper much now that Pop is gone. She says there isn't hardly any point. I notice more Kentucky Fried Chicken buckets in her refrigerator and fewer ham salad sandwiches being served for lunch.

Poppy died on August 14. As the last Thursday in November approaches, a year after his passing, I give Granny a call, but I don't want to. We haven't been close for quite some time, even before he died. After Frank and I split, I rebelled a little, dating a string of people my conservative town didn't approve of. I remember how my grandparents felt about Sheena being accepted into the church, and what the deacons would think if they knew she'd been invited to our home. I sensed it back then, but now I really know how wrong that was—their judgment, their ostracism of her. I knew a man I cared about would never be accepted if he had dark skin and cornrows, but that didn't make me consider it any less.

They wanted me to be with someone who looked the part of a Southern Baptist Republican, like Victor, so that I could grow into the role of the subservient little housewife like I was supposed to. I never brought anyone home to meet my family. Victor, the only one they would have accepted, wouldn't have come if I begged him, and it was probably better that way.

Maybe I was testing them with my choices. Maybe I just needed to know if they truly loved me, and in my mind, that was one way to learn the answer. I posted a photo of a man named Trey and myself on a date at Keeneland. It didn't take long for the news to make its way back to Gran and Pop. And I was right. When they found out about the "scandal," they called their preacher and asked the entire church to pray for me. I was humiliated.

They didn't speak to me for a long time after that—more than a year, I believe. It reinforced all the fears that I buried deep down inside. I just wanted to be loved unconditionally, but every time I did something "wrong" I was shunned, ignored, and gossiped about. It just proved, in my mind at least, that I had never really belonged with my family at all.

My random interactions with Victor over the years reinforced the judgment I felt from my grandparents. Full of shame, I always left our conversations feeling as though I was never good enough for him, like I would never be lucky enough for someone like him to love someone like me. Like the only person they'd feel worthy for me to bring home would be too embarrassed to be seen with me and *my* family.

Never, not once, did they have an actual conversation with me about how they felt about my dating choices. Never once did they ask my side of the story, or why I did what I did, said what I said, or felt what I felt. That was my entire life. And it hurt. Time softened it some, and Granny and I were speaking again by the time Poppy got sick.

"What time is Thanksgiving dinner this year? Want me to make anything?" I say when I finally build up the nerve to call her.

"Just come whenever you want, Kasey."

I don't understand.

"Is that what you're telling everyone? To come when they want?" I ask.

"Well, I reckon. I don't want to be an inconvenience," she says.

It is not about inconveniencing; it is about breaking our tradition.

"If everyone comes when they want, how can we be sure that we all eat together? What if Brother is hungry by lunch, and I'm not until later in the day?"

"Just come when you want. How's Maime?" she says, changing the subject. The dinner that only happened once a year and held our family together is now hanging on by a thread.

Poppy would have never stood for it. "Come when you want? Phooey!" He would have told her it was as dumb as tits on a bull. But he isn't here to make her toe the line—he isn't here to pick up the mess everyone made. He is gone, I am here, and it should feel like home, but it doesn't. Not anymore. And I blame Granny for that.

Frank's Clone—2014 to 2015

When you don't address problems in your life, they come back as clones. In 2015, I marry Jacob, Frank's Clone.

———

Pop is gone, and I find myself searching even harder for something or someone to fill that void inside my heart. I need stability again—I hurt for it.

Every now and again I communicate with Victor even though I know better. He meets a need of mine, to be desired, even if I know it's wrong.

Each time something bad happens I tell myself I haven't been good enough. I treated Frank like shit, and I deserve punishment for wanting more.

Maybe a deep connection with another human being is too much to ask for? And enough passion to light a room on fire is only made for the movies? I am being selfish, I guess, and loneliness is my punishment for that.

Sitting in the fifth row, stage left, at Sunday church service, I vow that if God brings me a man with a good heart, I will never do anything to take that love for granted. I want someone who is proud to stand by my side, one who is proud of me for being me.

I watch him play the guitar from the crowd. I listen to him sing and I'm drawn in—the music makes me feel something.

"Do you give guitar lessons?" I ask in a direct message on social media. I am hoping the question will open the door to a relationship, and it does.

One week passes, and we sit together in the back of the auditorium, playing Words with Friends on our cell phones while the preacher delivers his sermon.

This is my answered prayer. He is crazy about me—obsessed, even.

"Wanna go eat Chinese?" he asks.

"Uh, sure," I say while internally laughing.

God. I asked for a good heart, not a sophisticated palate.

After the first date, he never leaves; I think that's what I need, someone who will never leave. Someone who wants to be with me so badly that they'll do anything to make me happy. I've been searching for fulfillment for so long, and I think our relationship will give me that.

Laundry Basket Baby—2014

I work as a therapist for a large nonprofit agency doing in-home counseling services with children in rural south-central Kentucky. My office can be found in the trunk of my car, along with a suitcase full of toys and the necessary bug spray.

I learn a lot at this job, like the difference between a bed bug, a water bug, and a termite. I know what a baby deer looks like up close, thanks to the client who raises one in her living room. Thanks to this job, I am given the opportunity to recognize the slight variations of rabbit poop and Raisinets, and now I know not to touch anything brown lying on the floor.

I am a newish therapist, so I expect to get the hard cases. I take every bug and rodent in stride and focus on what I am there to do: help my clients have a better life. I am committed to them, and my desire to help transform their future is stronger than my need for comfort, so I stay.

I work in that job for years, despite a deeply rooted desire to create a business of my own. But it never seems to be the right time.

On a hot day, sometime before Halloween, I crave a cherry Icee from the snack bar at the mall.

"Jacob, can you take me to the mall for a slushie?" I ask.

A short time later, he's carrying the largest size they sell out to me.

It tastes good: so cold in my mouth. *Exactly what I need.*

Barely out of the parking lot, with a strength that I didn't know I had, I used my right arm to heave the drink across the dash of the car. SPLAT. I look up to see little red beads of ice covering my vehicle from the floor to the ceiling. He slams on the brake and shoves the car in park. We both turn and look at one another.

What have I done?

"What did you do?" he asks.

Great question.

I am silent. He is stunned.

I am ashamed. He is still stunned.

I am afraid. I am sick. I am irrational.

I am pregnant.

This isn't the first time I have felt like this.

Two little pink lines tell me all I need to know. They tell me that my life is about to change again, and this time I am excited about it. Jacob is excited, too, after he cleans up the Icee from the nooks and crannies of the car. He tells me he'll never leave me, and I believe him.

At twenty weeks, I drive to my OB appointment for a regular checkup, but less than five minutes into the exam, the look on my doctor's face tells me something is wrong.

"I need you to listen carefully. Go home, pack a bag, and be back at six in the morning, sharp. You'll be my first patient for surgery."

"What?" I ask.

"You're dilating. Your body is trying to go into labor. We have to stop it, or you'll lose your baby."

Again?

I walk out of the building in shock. *What did I do to deserve this?*

I do what I am told and show up for surgery bright and early the next morning. It is successful: it does what it was designed to do and keeps my baby alive. Now my time is spent on strict bed rest, with a makeshift bed frame, all because I must sell the only piddly one I have to pay the water bill.

I battle depression, loneliness, anger, and guilt the entire pregnancy. I strongly consider taking my own life, but I can't stand the thought of my daughter feeling alone like I do now. I am laid off from my job because I am unable to fulfill my duties. I am forced to file for bankruptcy because I can't work, and bills don't pay themselves.

I hit rock bottom.

My vehicle gets repossessed because I can't afford the payment. I watch in shame from inside my bedroom window as they haul it away. Lying there facing up at the popcorn ceiling, I make projections about the business I dream of owning, even though numbers terrify me. I calculate my risks but ask myself, *Can it get any worse?* Could I lose any more than I've already lost? At a time in my life when I should be overcome with joy, I'm instead consumed with fear. I can't help but worry that I'll lose my baby and not be able to afford the funeral.

Months pass, and when she takes her first breath, it is like *I* can finally breathe again. I am happy again for the first time since Pop died. Holding her makes me feel like I have a purpose. She makes me appreciate time differently. She teaches me that patience is vital, because that is what saved her life. She helps me to cherish every moment she stayed right where she belonged, with me.

I name her Lennon.

I sold everything I had of any value so that I could pay the electric bill, and by the time I bring her home from the hospital I must put my newborn baby girl in a laundry basket to sleep, because that's all I can afford. Watching her through the holes in the white plastic sleeping so soundly there gives me so much peace. It reminds me that a baby doesn't care where she sleeps. She is happy if she is warm with a belly full of milk and someone who loves her.

Even when Jacob and I later struggle to love each other, we love her more than anything in the world. I watch her smile and hope that she dreams of me one day—that she's proud of me, that she loves me even half as much as I love her.

Business—2017

I have done well for myself.

I started the mental health practice I dreamed about during all those days on bed rest. I poured my heart and soul into it. I told myself that this was the way to freedom and fulfillment. By its second year it grossed over a million dollars, and I am right about the freedom part.

After two years as an entrepreneur, a leader in the healthcare industry notices me and asks me to be a part of his consulting program. It's what I want to do. I want to teach others because that feels like part of who I am.

I fly to Michigan for his business owners' retreat celebrating the lost art of slowing down. It is my first business's second anniversary, and slowing down is not something I have even considered in those first couple of years. I know if I want to make a name for myself in the consulting world, I need to put myself *out* into the consulting world. This would be my debut.

⎯⎯⎯⎯

Northern Michigan is beautiful; it's everything people told me it would be. Clean, pristine, and pure. I sit at the Cherry Capital Airport in Traverse City, anxiously awaiting the other professionals that are here for a week of slowing down, too. The mere thought of social interaction takes a toll on me, though.

I sit huddled in a corner just like a cactus would, admiring my surroundings from a distance. I take everything in—careful not to get too close to anything or anyone. After about an hour, people start trickling in, and I watch them. I am interested. I've never met a group of entrepreneurs like these before.

I'm laser-focused on goals and desperate to succeed. In my mind, that means staying busy. Before I left home, I packed a *helluva* suitcase. I know it is supposed to be a S-L-O-W-D-O-W-N conference, but in my bag, I have every piece of paper I need to analyze my profit and loss statements for the month and complete the payroll that is due today. I tell myself that overworking is the price of success. The fact that I sit here with a five-inch stack of reports means that I must love my business more than everyone else loves theirs. I am more dedicated, more involved, and more determined.

Secretly, I never relax. My body might try, but my brain hardly ever slows down. I'm a control freak; I know this about myself—but I also know that's what my business needs from me. A big ole type-A, batshit-crazy, overfunctioning control freak. But when I see how chill everyone else is, I quickly change my game plan. I can't be the only one over here doing payroll. I need to look a little less obvious, and I need to do it quickly! I'm not going to let any of these people know how neurotic I am.

No! I am going to sit here and make them think I am calm, cool, and collected—like I got it all together, because I totally do. Totally.

I *am* a real-deal professional. I wear black slip-on flats or pumps with pantsuits. Where I come from, that's how you gauge one's credibility or at least their ability to achieve success—how they dress or how much they spent to rebuild their vintage hotrod. Here are the qualifying questions:

1. Did you brush your hair and not just the part you can see in the mirror? *Check.*
2. Did you apply enough mascara to not look dead? *Check!*
3. Are you wearing your best suit from JCPenney with the extra poufy shoulder pads? *Check!!*

Voilà! You're a professional! *I* am a professional. I have completed all those things. I even have a fancy Michael Kors leather work bag for which I saved nearly six months to buy. I am on my best behavior, smiling politely, trying not to be the loudest in that room, but not totally invisible either.

A rumbling sound creeps toward me like a hurricane rolling out from baggage claim. One hand holding the suitcase haphazardly, and the other arm moving like a Weed Eater—gaining momentum to take everyone out around her. Wild and bouncing curls loosely contained by a ponytail holder move from side to side as she walks. She's totally in the moment, just taking it all in. She waves to strangers, points at cute babies, and scans the room in a way that is certainly the opposite of me.

That woman doesn't have a care in the world. I see her acknowledge the crowd as it begins to assemble around her.

"What's up, fuckers!" she says loudly.

I grab onto the arm of the chair I am sitting in with my left hand and cover my mouth with my right.

Mouth open.

Eyes fixed.

My ears zero in on her every word.

Did that woman really just say fuck? I don't even say that word. That is a bad word. A dirty word. Like, a really, really, bad word. I said "frigging" one time when I was in eighth grade, and my mom smacked my mouth hard enough to make me blink three times and then shoved a bar of soap in it. But *that wild woman* said it right there in front of the entire airport. *She must be one of those northern people.*

Wonder what's it like to be like that?

To give zero Fs?

To carry yourself in a way that makes no apologies for who and what you are. To myself, and only to myself, while barely moving my lips so no one can see, I whisper the word *fuck.* I need to see how it feels coming out of my mouth.

F-u-u-a-a-a-c-k.

Oh dang.

I say it again.

F-u-u-a-a-a-c-k.

Yep, not the word for me.

But it seems natural for her.

Based on what she's told us all in the last five minutes, I have come to learn she's a couples counseling–loving, external-processing, noisemaking free spirit who is at the same conference as me to grow her business. She is curious, loud, and overly friendly, *not* just like me. She is everything I am not. She scares me.

It takes another hour before our host arrives and loads everyone into the full-sized yellow school bus waiting for us outside the airport. I cautiously make my way up the big plastic-coated steps. I look for a seat, careful not to impose on anyone's personal space along the way. I spot an empty one in the back of the bus, and I make a beeline. I get the luxury of choosing the spot far away from all the people and avoid the awkward chitchat I suspect might be coming. But, to my surprise, Tara is also one of the first people on the bus, which means she gets dibs on a perfect seat, too.

I see her head pop up from the stairs, and I hear her making her way down the aisle. I slump down so she doesn't see me. She bumps each aisle-sitting person with her bag, her arm, and her flip flops. Each time she offers up a quick *oopsie*, makes a joke, and keeps on walking. Thankfully there are enough seats for everyone to have their own and enough space in between for my own personal comfort. My optimism is short-lived when I realize that in Tara's hunt for the perfect seat, her eyes are locked in on the same one as mine, and she isn't slowing down.

Oh no.

She's getting closer to me.

Is she going to sit by me? Is she going to call me a fucker? What am I going to say? How will I handle that? I don't even cuss.

I am nervously holding my breath. One, two, three, four, five. Tara plops herself, her bag, and her big ole personality down right. Next. To. ME.

"Whazzzzupp! You're Kasey from Ken-tu-cky, right?" she says with the worst southern drawl I've ever heard. "I'm Tara, and we're going to be best friends!"

———

I want to focus on my business, but Jacob's texting is relentless. I can tell he is spiraling. Tara is the one to catch me crying in the bathroom and asks a question that I wish I didn't have to answer.

"Are you okay?" she asks.

Jacob is threatening to divorce me because of this trip. I'm not giving him enough attention. I'm focusing too much on my business, and I received an innocent message from one of my best friends telling me he saw I was on Lake Michigan, and he "wished he was there." To Jacob, back home reading my messages from my child's iPad, this clearly means I'm having an affair.

"I'm not cheating on him," I say.

I hide in the bathroom for extended periods of time, take long walks outside alone, and sneak away from meetings for enough privacy to argue with him about why I can't talk to him all day. I feel pulled in so many directions. Tend to my marriage, tend to my professional relationships, tend to my business, tend to my children, and try to do it with equal amounts of effort. Give each one 100 percent, all the time, no questions asked.

Impossible.

Part of me understands where Jacob is coming from. It is the first time we have been away from one another overnight since the first time he slept over. I have been bedridden nearly all of our relationship, meaning he knew where I was all the time. I had little to no autonomy and up until now I have relied on him for so much. We have become terribly codependent, and now it is clear that our relationship is unhealthy.

"He's so angry with me, and nothing I say or do helps," I say. I agree to never speak to my friend again, but he's still upset. I promise to never go on a trip without him again, but he's still mad. I basically promise him everything if he will just calm down. My insides are hurting, and my body is in dire dysregulation.

"Find your own ride home from the airport," he says.

I sob uncontrollably in the fetal position behind a large column at the airport awaiting my flight back home, while Tara, who is mostly still a stranger, sits by my side.

"He's going to leave me," I say.

Just when I thought everything was starting to fall into a normal routine and a normal life, this happens.

"I should have just stayed home. I have no business flying to another state, trying to meet other professionals. I don't need to grow my career, anyway," I say.

She doesn't say anything. She listens. The thought of telling anyone, especially my family, causes my body to shudder—they'll be so disappointed. Lennon will be another child from a broken home. I can't breathe from the weight of the shame I feel for wanting more—all because I went after a dream.

A missed flight and an extra layover later, I move down the escalator toward baggage claim, fully prepared to hitchhike home. I haven't heard a word from him since the last time he hung up on me back at the layover in Detroit. As I slowly raise my eyes up to meet the ground, I see his tennis shoes.

He hands me a bouquet of roses. We never speak about it again.

Red Fold-Up Chair—2018

They say you may stray, but you'll always end up close to where you started.

In the fall of 2018, the trees are still ripe, and I have entered another season. Still firmly attached to their creator, the leaves appear to enjoy their time there. Twenty-four hours a day, they peer from the eighty-foot cliff overlooking the delicate ripple of Lake Cumberland. Securely witnessing the brave souls walking out onto the ledge of Needle Point, staring down, testing their courage, they lie where I spent many summer days as a high school senior. They glisten from the morning dew and cast deep shadows on the evening's hillside. They are like flies on the walls; they hear and see everything on Edgewater Drive.

I have so many memories of the Old Man and me going for drives and daydreaming about the houses nestled back off the main roads. *What must it be like to live in one of those?* I asked him questions about how much they cost, how much the land impacted the value, and if he ever thought I would live somewhere like that. All the while dreaming of what my house would look like one day. I like to believe he, too, has an admiration for architecture and an appreciation for the things that intrigue his daughter, but he never says much more than what I prompt him to. He is a man of few words, unless of course you get him talking about the good ole days back when he was in the service; then he won't stop.

He has lived in the same place for as long as I can remember, right down the road from where I sit on Edgewater. Although it doesn't have a view of the water, from Dad's place the trained nose can smell it.

We gravitate toward the lake on our weekend drives, even if it is nothing more than to catch a glimpse of the color changes or just to see how many boats are putting in. I stare out the window as I sip my orange soda and tear away at my beef jerky. He picks up the same things from Slate Branch gas station every weekend before we head out on our adventure. A cigarette burns, ashes fly in the cab from the breeze, and his elbow is propped up, sticking partially out the window while we drive. He looks happy.

It doesn't take too long, about as much time for me to finish my jerky before I hear him say, "You wanna drive?"

Of course I want to drive. He pitstops at the same subdivision, the one down the road on the right, with only a few houses and mostly open lots.

"What gear's it in?" I ask.

"Neutral," he pipes back at me. "How many times do I have to tell you it goes in neutral when we switch seats?"

I know this already.

And off we go.

I don't know if the Old Man ever thinks about the houses as I drive or dreams of owning one for himself, or if he is content living side by side with his mom and dad in the little trailer he continues to add on to. I don't know if he pays much attention to the changing colors of the leaves, but I know he pays a lot of attention to me in the driver's seat, and I like that.

Our little weekend tradition carried me through my teen years and, now, on into adulthood. Whenever I need to think, I take to the roads, windows down, wind hitting me in the face, and Smashing Pumpkins, an American alternative rock band, blaring through the speakers.

In the fall of 2018, I finally feel like I am doing okay at life. I have overcome professional challenges, personal struggles, and financial hardships. It hasn't been easy, but I am on the other side of it, and for that, I am thankful. I bought my first house just a year ago; I have two beautiful girls and two dogs, more than anyone could ask for. My mental health business is doing well, and my consulting firm is up and coming. I can catch a glimpse of the water from that first house bought since coming out of bankruptcy.

As I numbly scroll through Facebook, a house pops up for sale in a familiar location. It is a seven-acre lot that Jacob and I looked at once upon a time. We didn't buy it then because the land was already so expensive. I worried that I wouldn't be able to afford to build a house. Instead, I purchased something already built and much more affordable. Looking at that seven-acre lot now, there is something magnificent on it.

My dream home. It is love at first sight.

I hop in my Suburban and head down the familiar road toward the lake. Windows down as far as they go so I can smell the air, I slowly maneuver through my neighborhood, and turn left down a country road less than three hundred feet from where my dad and I used to go for drives. I venture past a subdivision I remember being built. I pass a trailer park on the left that I rode my moped through as a kid.

I take a hard right, and a fiery sunset blinds me from the west. Like all Kentucky evenings, deep, beautiful, and meaningful, it makes a bold statement. It's getting late and what was left of the sun reflects on a little oblong-shaped pond dotted with a few ducks and one baby cow catching a quick bath before nightfall.

The scene reminds me of why I still live here in Kentucky.

Up the hill, around a sharp curve, and down a steep descent, I drive under a rainbow arch of oak trees before the sky opens. There it is, Needle Point sitting confidently to my right in all its glory, the tourist attraction that all the northern folks come to see. The ripples in the water bring an instant sense of calm over me, and when my eyes wander left, I stop the vehicle and put it in park. I don't take my eyes off it, as my fingers instinctively open the driver's side door.

Left foot, right foot, road. Right there in the middle of the street, I stand staring at the structure on top of the hill. I come face to face with what feels like my childhood dreams becoming a potential reality.

It is just a house made of brick, stone, metal, and a ton of glass, but when I see it, it becomes more than that. I need to get closer, but it is still under construction. I hear a voice in my head say, "You wanna drive, Little'n?"

"I sure do, Old Man," I say aloud as an ornery smirk crosses my face. I get back behind the wheel and make my ascent to the top of the long driveway and the house's entrance.

There is no one there. Just me and the drywall dust, but the moment I walk through the front door, the feeling I had down in the middle of the road is validated. Before me is a panoramic view of the water, virtually unobstructed. A pontoon moves slowly around the outline of the shore, and a fishing boat flies around the corner, probably looking for the cove. The boat ramp we used to fish from as a kid sits directly in front of me. It is like watching my childhood from a much better vantage point.

Energy pulls me forward. The chalky white footprints follow me from the front door, across the living room and kitchen, to the porch, where I stand in awe.

The front porch is massive. Teak wood on the ceiling, lights, and ceiling fans, it is big enough for at least three designated living areas. I picture an outdoor dining table to my left, with a grill where I will tend to baby back ribs and drink German grapefruit beer. I envision an outdoor living room set to put in the middle, perfect for catching my body so I can get lost in the sunsets. I can see a porch swing to the right swaying away those long days at work. I can see it all, all it could be, even in its unfinishedness.

But I don't have any of that yet. This isn't even my house, but it feels like it should be my *view*—my sunset and my water. It feels like it *could* be mine; it could be a significant part of my future. I believe that I can create the life, any life that I want. I just need clarity to do it. Staring across the property, my eyes land in the water, taking me right back to my childhood yet again: the drives with my dad, the meetups at the lake with friends, the secret place I used to go when I needed time to think. It brought me back to everything I used to feel.

Joy.

I'm lost in thought and can't say for sure how long I stand there.

Wait.

I take off toward the front door and open the back hatch of my vehicle. I grab the red fold-up chair that I use for watching Maime's soccer games. I position it in my favorite spot on the porch, the one in front of the bedroom. I sit down softly and inhale.

This is my porch now.

With no distractions, I watch the water until the sun finally tucks itself behind the tree line. The dropping sun reminds me it is time to go home, but I leave the chair on *my* porch. I know I'll be back.

In the months following, I crunch numbers like nobody's business. Is this house even possible? How much more money do I need? How much more do I need to work? Days and weeks pass, and I learn I am pregnant with my third child, which means even more to consider. The move, the change, the money . . . Am I crazy?

I don't tell Jacob because the idea feels too far out of reach. *I need to keep this little gem to myself, at least for now.* Also, if he or anyone else knows I am going back to that porch as often as I do, they'd have my sanity evaluated. There is nothing wrong with dreaming, right?

I take books there and read. I visit at different times of the day to get a different view of the sunset. I stand in the bedroom and look out the window, imagining what it would feel like to wake up to this each morning. I stand at the spot made for a stove, look out the window, and imagine what it would be like to eat a steak cooked to perfection and drink a glass of bourbon with this view.

We all have our thing. This is mine.

It is midday on a Saturday, and I sneak off for a little bit to read some Donald Miller and listen to the boats. I sit in the red fold-up chair and prop my feet up on the wire railing. By this time, it is late spring, and I am pretty good and pregnant. That's right, instead of getting divorced, Jacob and I decide to have another child.

It isn't all that comfortable, but the view trumps the pain of my little Thayer Bear kicking my left rib. With my book propped up on my growing belly, I hear a vehicle coming down the hill through the rainbow trees. I try to shrink down and pretend to be invisible. After all, this is not my house, at least not *technically.*

I turn my head and take my legs off the railing. I put my head down, I wait for them to pass, but they don't. I hear their engine slow, but I'm afraid to look. I fight the urge to look. Like a small child, I think, *They can't see me if I can't see them.* I stay hunkered down.

My worst-case scenario is confirmed when I hear the vehicle coming up the driveway, rattling muffler and all. Do I pretend to be looking at the house as a potential buyer? Do I hide in the bathroom, lock the door, or jump off the porch?

My heart races, but I am paralyzed by fear. The front door opens, and the windows shake when it closes. I feel the footsteps ruffle the house as they move toward me.

Play it cool, Kasey. You've talked your way out of much worse situations than this. Don't sweat. Act normal.

I can smell him before I see him. *Marlboros.*

"What are you doing here!" we both say in tandem.

"What the hell?" we both say again.

We both chuckle.

"That's one helluva view," he says as he props his hands on the porch railing, flicking ashes off into the grass. "You should buy it."

I know why he is here, but I ask just to see what he says. He still likes to go on drives, too, and he discovered this house on one of them. He has an appreciation for dreaming just like me. Now I know the answer to the question I had when I was a kid: Does Dad dream?

He looks over at my red fold-up chair and chuckles. I know what he is thinking. That is something he would do, too.

I take this serendipitous meeting as a sign. My dad likes this house, too. He found me here, doing the very same thing he was doing, admiring its beauty. I wonder if he's ever sat in the red fold-up chair when he visits.

"That yours?" he says as he walks toward the door. "Sits kinda crooked."

———

I move into the house nearly three months later, right before the birth of my son. I sit down on my brand-new outdoor couch, positioned in the middle of the porch just as I had imagined. This time I don't have to worry about anyone coming up the driveway and telling me I don't belong there. This is my porch now. My view. My water. My house. My dream.

My Voice–2020

Aside from the fact that my family life is and probably always will be dysfunctional, my professional one is going well.

———————

Outside, the wind kisses the branches and tickles the window. The sun still peeks through the palm trees as if they're keeping an eye on me. In the distance, ripples dance in the pond where Sherman the alligator likes to sunbathe. I bought the beach house just a few months ago at the onset of the COVID-19 pandemic, and this is one of my first experiences on Fripp Island as a homeowner.

I brought Maime on the trip with me because she's old enough to occupy herself while I work.

"I'm only here to write," I tell her. "I probably won't be much fun."

It is my writing coach's last virtual editing retreat of the year, and I need to finish my manuscript.

I make good progress, weaving what AJ calls Kaseyisms into each section. It's the last day, and the pressure is on to put the finishing touches on my last chapter. I perch on the lounge chair in the living room, my computer propped up on the arm. I glance at the itinerary for the day, and I see that I will be sharing a part of my book with the other students. I'm excited, but a little nervous, too. I worked so hard on the last chapter, digging deep, channeling my southern roots, and keeping my beloved Granny Lillie, to whom I dedicated the chapter, in mind the entire time.

She's been on my mind a lot the closer I get to finishing the book. I love writing about her childhood.

As I write about her, I let go of everything, including the pain, both past and present. I become so lost in the story that I nearly forget I am writing a business book. I write what is in my heart and let my mind remember her as well as everyone else who has played a special role in my life.

"You're up," AJ says.

I begin to read the chapter aloud, slowly. I sink down into the words, linger in the feelings, and when I finally look up from the page, I see tears in their eyes.

"Kasey Compton," Laura, her dean of students, says.

And that is enough. That's all that needs to be said—all I need to hear.

I feel it. The validation, the triumph, the prickle of my own tears emerging from the corners of my eyes. I wish Maime hadn't gone to the beach looking for shells. I wish she could be here, experiencing this incredible moment with me. I hope she, too, will be proud of me when she reads it.

"Fannie Flagg, when did you get here?" AJ says.

I smile, breathless.

"Kasey Compton, my dear," she says as she tugs on her glasses. Her eyes are cloudy, and her voice is soft.

"Welcome to authorship. *You*, my dear, have found your voice."

I pack the car with our luggage. It feels strange carrying a much lighter load with it being just me and Maime this time. She sits as far in the back as she can, enjoying the privacy of the third row. We make it off the island and into Beaufort County in about forty-five minutes.

The traffic starts to slow. There's congestion as we approach the line to cross the drawbridge. Down below is a barge, just like the ones I see nearly every time I'm here. I take this opportunity to slow down and admire the Lowcountry and all of its beauty.

From the perspective of the bridge, it's as if the world has slowed, too. Unbeknownst to it, an intangible object, this bridge is a gift to all of us, especially me. One that allows me a chance to admire the birds, the flickers in the water, and my daughter in the back seat. I turn up the music playing quietly on the radio, roll down the windows, and open the sunroof to let in as much sun possible. I pull as much air from my lungs as I can from my belly and in through my nose. I exhale slowly and start to sing.

My voice.

I know what AJ meant about finding it, but I wonder if she knows it means more to me. Finding my author voice feels like an even greater significance, much in the same way as becoming a mother did. It was as if I finally connected to an untapped piece of me, one that was walled up, waiting on me to let down the drawbridge.

Every place I have been, everything I have experienced—my family, my struggles, my insecurities—they all mean something now. Everything together makes up my voice—it is a part of me. I think about how my voice resembles the person I am, how I've struggled to find her. How I felt so insecure, never wanting others to hear it. Fearful of being judged, criticized, and rejected, I've been metaphorically silent for years.

The bridge starts to lower, and the traffic inches forward. I can't help but think about how it feels this time; crossing the bridge to go back home is different now, maybe because I am different. Maybe it's because, in part, I've let something down inside of my own heart, allowing for movement, progress, and hope.

I peek into my rearview to see Maime, eyes fixated on the water, a smile spread across her face. She is singing, too. I watch joy move over her freckled cheeks and pour from her mouth with each note that plays on the radio. I feel *her* joy wash over me like I am feeling it for the first time myself.

She sees me, there in this moment watching her, and she stops. Her body language changes, her eyes dart downward, and her lips stop moving all together. It is almost as if she is ashamed of the joy she feels.

What a familiar feeling it is. One I have felt so many times around my own mother. One that caused me to silence my voice, in fear that my own happiness would cause her more pain. One that made me feel guilty for doing well, being happy, or being me. A feeling so familiar that I never want my daughter to feel it again.

The Conversation—June 2021

Sometimes, things feel like they come out of nowhere, but they don't. They've been brewing, festering under the surface for longer than we realize. We're just too busy to notice.

Kelsey, an employee of my practice since 2019, is an acquaintance. We go on an occasional birthday outing together with the girls from the office, an annual business retreat or two, but never anything more.

The first serious conversation we ever had happened about three weeks before the book launch.

"Can I talk to you?" she asks while standing in the door to my office.

I know what this means.

Resignation.

Anytime I'm asked that question, someone's about to give me their two-week notice. I brace myself and hesitantly say, "Sure. Come on in."

With her in my office, I am oddly nervous.

I've never been this close to her before. I've never been alone with her before. Ever since our first interaction at the employee entrance, I have felt an urge to avoid her.

She makes me curious in a reckless kind of way. Her personality is contagious. The feelings seem dangerous, so up until now, I have pretended they didn't exist.

I am out of my element around her, and that scares me. I am drawn to her deeply, in a way that feels different from anyone else.

For two years I've thought about her randomly, like what her natural hair color is, if she notices me avoiding her, and about her northern accent that makes most words that come out of her mouth sound funny. I think about how she puts on a tough exterior, but underneath she must be sensitive. I don't know what to make of these thoughts; I can't tell anyone about them, so I tell myself to stop.

Sweat beads up under my arms, and I become self-conscious of my appearance. *Can she smell me?*

I sit across the room from her, waiting nervously to hear what she needs. Her eyes are serious and intentional, but she is smiling. Her foot tapping creates a melody in the room—one that I can feel rush through the blood of my body with every beat of my heart. Like an awkward dance, she moves from the wingback chair to the doorframe and back to the chair again before she ever gets out her first word. She is nervous.

I notice her hands. How her fingers move around and around a piece of straw casing. They look soft but strong, nonetheless. I breathe heavily, but oddly enough, her nervousness calms me. Her presence in my office makes me happy; it always has, but I can't say why.

"Therapy," she says finally, coming to her point abruptly, as if she doesn't say it now, maybe she won't. "Who do you recommend?"

"It depends. Is it for you?" I ask.

"I mean, nothing's wrong with me," she says. "I just need to sort some things out."

Sort some things out?

Why do you make me so nervous?

Maybe I'm the one who needs to sort things out.

I try to keep a strong poker face, sure not to let her see how much I want to know more. The last thing I want to do is embarrass her, but I am honored that she trusts me enough with this question.

"There's only one person I would see around here," I say. "I'll email you her contact info."

But that's not what I want to say. I want to ask her questions. I have so many questions.

"Are you okay?" I blurt out impulsively.

It's almost as if I'm outside of my body. I watch how her lips cover her teeth and how she holds her mouth open longer when she thinks. I notice her fingers, how her nails are flat and round on the ends, kind of like Poppy's were. I imagine her toes must look the same. I find myself lost in her, listening to her talk but feeling the connection to her in my body at the same time.

"Not really, but thanks for the recommendation," she says on her way out of my office.

I say nothing.

I feel everything.

"Hey, you know you can talk to me, right?" I say.

She smiles.

"Same."

There *is* something upsetting her. She's looking for something, help, maybe. I don't want to push too far, but I don't want her to think I don't care either. This type of exchange is out of the norm for us, so it's hard for me to navigate.

I don't know what to do.

I have this desire to be close to her, and I don't mean sexually. I wonder what it would be like to hug her, what it would feel like for her to hug me back. I want to know how she smells and if she wears men's cologne. I want to know why I have these feelings. I want to talk to someone about it, too, but I tell myself I can't, because it is forbidden; she is forbidden.

I want to know why she's hurting. I want to help her. I need to know what *it* is. I think I already do, but my mind searches for the answer.

I'm distracted.

I'm distant.

I'm consumed with emotion.

And all those years I felt ignored, looked over, and insignificant—like I was invisible, *now* is when someone decides to pay attention.

Now, Jacob notices something about me is different.

The Fight—July 2021

Tension all around is high. I'm being accused. I'm not being heard. I am being suffocated. Among other things.

I tolerate the severity of it for five grueling days. It is the longest and most unsettling almost week of my life.

The details are too hard to share. It's not something I can even put on my timeline.

It's bad.

His reactions and his suspicion about Kelsey have shown me everything I need to know about him, about myself, and about what my life is going to look like if I continue denying the brutal truth about our relationship.

Five days after the first fight, I file for divorce. Nearly a month later, I publish my book.

But now I just want out.

Out of the chaos.

Out of the uncertainty.

Out of the obligation.

Out of the cage.

Just out.

Intimacy–August 2021

The feelings come in waves. Most of the time I can't make them stop or anticipate when they're going to start. They show up unexpectedly, and the more I
allow myself to feel things, the more *she* is top of mind.

"Are you nervous?" I ask when she comes back to my office one day after
the launch.

"Do I look nervous?"

"You're answering my question with a question," I say.

"Am I?"

We laugh.

"You've always made me nervous," she admits, grinning. "You are kind of
intimidating."

"I know." I flip a tendril of hair that has fallen loose from my messy bun sar-
castically. This is the first moment I've forgotten about the hell I'm in.

She laughs like she knows exactly what I'm doing. It doesn't sound flirtatious,
not like other girls laugh around people they like. It is her real laugh, genuine
and soft, but it makes my stomach flip. I want to keep the laughing going, the
conversation going, everything going so it never stops. I have completely forgotten
why she is here again in the first place. I am only thinking about keeping this easy
rhythm as long as I can.

At some point the conversation turns, and neither of us wants to bring it back. It is 2 PM on a Thursday, and usually my head would be full of everything I need to do so I can enjoy a quiet Friday at home, but after we start talking, I forget everything.

Hopes, dreams, music, passion, possibilities—we talk about it all.

I ask her what she wants out of life and if she is happy. As a light comes in from the window behind her, enough to cast a shadow on her cheek, I see her differently—beyond the surface. Her eyes are now an even lighter green, a color I have never seen on her before. They avoid me, and I wonder why. When a tear rolls down her face, I see that she's vulnerable. She is strong, but sitting in front of me, she is exposed and brave. So I soften. I wonder what it is about my question that causes her pain. I am sorry. I am worried. I feel this unrelenting need to protect her. To understand her. So I encourage her to tell me more. And this time she does.

"I feel stuck. I've been going through the motions for a while now," she says. "I don't know what I want in the next five years, the next five days, or the next five minutes."

She has never given herself permission to dream.

She has no idea the meaning her life holds. She doesn't know how to live when the possibilities are unrestricted. She has no idea how special she is.

But *I* do.

"Can I tell you something?" I ask.

She nods.

"Mirror—it's like—" I stop to gather my thoughts. "It's like you are a mirror to me—one that I have refused to look into for the last decade of my life."

She leans forward, closer toward me.

"Everything you just told me was everything I needed to see in myself," I continue. "We have more in common than I thought."

She is so open that I figure I can be honest with her, too. I don't know the full extent of what my thoughts and feelings mean, I just know that I am not alone in them.

She sneaks a peek at her phone as a quick buzz brings us back to reality. She rises from the chair, hastily rubbing her face to rid herself of any lingering emotion. "I gotta go," she says.

I listen intently to her footsteps as they move toward the door. Hands on the frame, she pauses. Looking over her shoulder, dead in my eye, she smiles again.

She is beautiful.

I close my eyes because I can't bear to watch her leave. I don't want her to go. Ever. I listen to her footsteps move away until they abruptly stop.

Come back.

I can't explain it. I don't know what I would say if she does, but it feels good with her nearby. It feels safe, and not just with my physical being, but with my heart.

I want more time. I want someone to trust me the way that she just trusted me. I want someone who will listen to me the way she does, accept me the way she does, care for me the way I know she can. I don't know if it's her, or someone else someday, but I know I want more than I have had.

I hear her footsteps pick up again—but instead of closer, they become fainter and fainter with every second that passes. Before I know it, I am left breathless, sitting on my couch, lost in a moment.

Is this what real communication feels like?

It is messy, scary, and raw, but I love every single second of it. I breathe it all in, every word, every sound, every light, and every shadow—I let it consume me. I let myself marinate in it.

It has never been this way. My parents, partners, even my closest friends have never been so open with me. I can't remember the last time I felt so . . . *seen?*

The situation is unfamiliar and uncomfortable, but I don't run from it. Regardless of the outcome, wherever it takes me, I'm here for it. And in that moment with Kelsey, I am gentle because that's what she needs, that's what she deserves.

Maybe if my mom had been healthier when I was small, conversations like this would have happened more often. Maybe my friendships would have been stronger, and my marriages would have lasted. Maybe if someone would have modeled vulnerability for me at a young age, this conversation wouldn't have rattled me like it did—maybe it wouldn't have felt so unfamiliar.

My therapist encourages me to think about the needs of my Inner Child— what she needed when I was a little girl and what she still needs. I didn't realize how complex those needs were because I never experienced it. But now that I have,

I *know* that she needs to see and be seen by others. She needs vulnerability. She needs love.

She needs *intimacy*.

And so, at thirty-seven years old, I have my first *intimate* experience, and it's with a woman. It is with Kelsey.

Pink Dress—December 2021

"Kasey Renee," Granny says, "You better make sure they bury me in that pink dress hanging in my closet."

"Granny, you've told me this at least one hundred times. That's not something I could forget even if I wanted to."

"Mommy—what's Granny talkin' bout? What pink dress?" Lennon asks.

"Honey, don't pay Granny no mind," I say. "She isn't going anywhere anytime soon."

I fluff Lennon's hair, pat on her head, and smile over at Granny sipping on a plastic hospital pitcher full of ice water.

"You stubborn old mule, you'll outlive us all," I tell her.

She smiles and reaches out to touch my hand. I catch her wink at Lennon as I turn to walk out of the room.

———

Three weeks later, I get the call.

"She's gone, Little'n," Dad tells me. "The nursing home just called and told us to get up there."

I hurt for her, but I hurt for my kids more. They loved their Granny, especially Len.

"How old was Granny?" she asks when I tell her.

"Ninety-one years old, honey," I reply. "She lived a long life."

"What was wrong with her?"

There's no way I can tell her how bad the bed sores were underneath the hospital gown she wore day and night. She doesn't need to know the toll the falls had on her while she insisted on living alone. I feel guilty for thinking of her as my Big Granny because she has nearly withered away to nothing. Lennon doesn't need to hear that her kidneys shut down and her liver was no longer functioning.

"She was old, honey."

"She's in heaven now, isn't she, Mommy?"

I nod and smile at her sad little face. She has tears in her big blue eyes. "It's okay to cry—I know you're sad, but Granny is at home with Poppy now, and that's where she wants to be."

"And with Jesus?"

I nod.

She scoots from my lap and walks toward the front door of the house. With one hand gripping the handle, she turns and looks over her shoulder at me as if she forgot something.

"Oh! Mommy. Hey, don't forget to bury Granny in her pink dress."

"I won't forget, baby. I won't."

She remembered, so how could I forget.

Honesty—November 2021

"Has anything come up for you this week?" my therapist asks.

It's only been fourteen days since our last session, seven since I finished drawing out my life. Everything is happening so fast. Of course, there have been things that have come up for me. *How am I supposed to answer that?*

I have been worried, sad, and afraid of the Big Things happening in my life. I mean, I feel better that I'm sorting it all out, but it's hard. It's like I'm dealing with the present while processing the past, laying my heart on the line to piece together a better future. Not to mention holding down five businesses, three kids, and the unexpected new feelings for a woman.

When you spend your entire adult life shutting off feelings and repressing memories, they come back in a flood. It's overwhelming. And now, here I am, thinking about how I can unpack it all in the next sixty minutes for my therapist.

"Let me think," I say.

I spent approximately three hours of the week crying in my closet so my children wouldn't see me. I spent every moment that I stood in front of the mirror—washing my hands, putting on my clothes, brushing my teeth or my hair—trying to recognize myself for the first time in a long time. I spent at least thirty minutes a day in the bathroom, sitting on the toilet, fully clothed (mind you) just for peace and quiet. I spent hours researching places to take my kids so they could forget the miserable situation their dad and I put them in. I even considered taking them to Disney World, and when that becomes an option, I know I'm desperate.

"A few things," I tell her. "Drawing out my life has brought up even more memories, more connections, and some have been hard to accept."

"Tell me more."

"Last week, you said that I needed to raise my standards and form a new baseline for love. But here's the thing. I don't know how to tell when something is a red flag or if it's just something that happens because we're human."

Hearing my own words spoken aloud, I make another realization.

I don't trust myself.

I am finally being honest. I have stopped trying to make myself believe that my life is fine, because it isn't. I've spent the last decade overcompensating with forgiveness and grace because I gave Frank none, and I know how that feels. Now I don't know when to leave, so I stay in unhealthy relationships because it's easier. I don't have boundaries or standards, for that matter, because I don't love myself.

"Do you feel guilty for wanting what you need?" she asks.

I do.

"I have a question for you," she says. I brace myself. "All the *Little Things* you told me that happened in your relationship with Jacob you said were not divorce-worthy. But to me, they *were*. Why were you so resistant to moving forward with separation back then when all those Little Things happened?"

"You mean the first time he came to my house and stole money from me?" I giggle. "It was Frank," I continue. "I fought so hard to make it work because I didn't want to prove Frank right. When he looked at me and said I'd never be satisfied—that I was incapable of a successful relationship—I didn't want him to be right, so I stayed to prove him wrong."

"What about Victor?" she says out of the blue. "Were you thinking about him, too?"

"Probably a little. I wanted to prove him wrong as well. I wanted to prove everyone wrong."

"What did you have to prove to *him*?"

I settle in and breathe through my feelings. "Victor and I had a lot of conversations throughout the years. He knew me when I was poor—he knew me at my lowest. When I started dating Jacob, Victor wanted to see me again, of course. I wanted closure, so I agreed."

I lived in a tiny brick box, sparsely decorated with hand-me-down furniture, with a kitchen that was barely functional. But Maime and I had a roof over our heads, and at that point, it was good enough. I was too embarrassed to let him see it, but I was about to end a ten-year stint of cat and mouse with a man that I believed was too good for me, so I let him in for the last time.

Emotions swoop in my body like he is standing before me again, our faces meeting through the screen door sometime after midnight. That's the only time he'd see me after all, when no one was watching—when he wouldn't be judged for being interested in a single mom who didn't come from money. *Trailer trash*, he called me a couple times after a few too many glasses of whiskey.

"Victor already knew that I was seeing Jacob, but he didn't care. I told him I was happy and that I never wanted to see him again."

With Jacob, at least, I would never have to live in a game of cat and mouse, and I would not have to fear that he would leave.

Victor hurt my heart. With every interaction, I felt smaller and smaller. He did this for nearly a decade, but I kept going back, entertaining a conversation or an email each time one came my way. But I was done doing that. It took too much from me, and by the time I met Jacob, I barely had anything left of myself.

"Once I cut that cord with Victor, it was over. I married Jacob a year after we had Lennon, and rarely ever thought about him again," I say.

"Except when you were trying to talk yourself into staying in your marriage. Then you told yourself it could be worse, right? Like how it was with Victor?"

"I guess so," I say.

At least Jacob was nice to me. His words didn't cut like Victor's did.

I was a shell of a person when Jacob came along. I was broken, confused, and empty. I accepted his shortcomings and turned a blind eye to the red flags because I wanted to pretend that they did not exist. Perhaps I even thought I wasn't worthy of someone free of flags.

The Little Things I experienced felt irrelevant in the grand scheme of things, but they weren't, and now I know they aren't irrelevant at all. They are the true tellin's of a person's heart, their intentions, and their motivations, but you have to choose to see them.

I realize now how much of an impact my conversations with Frank had on me. I didn't under any circumstances want him to watch me fail. I spent a lifetime attaching myself to outcomes, which has controlled me. Regardless of what the day-to-day looks like, if Jacob and I were still married, Frank couldn't say, *I told you so.*

"That's what's kept me there. That's why I accepted the lack of internal fulfillment because I didn't want Frank to be right."

I became laser-focused on success, and life became so much easier and more predictable with my blinders on, when I didn't feel. I could convince myself I wasn't always on the verge of losing someone I love. I felt more control over my life when I didn't live in the moment, when I always had a "next step" on my list.

I wasn't lying in the driveway feeling the leftover heat from the day's sun seeping through the concrete, watching the stars, or sitting on the porch listening to the deer in the trees. I wasn't playing music and dancing with my baby boy in my living room before bedtime. I wasn't having conversations with my daughter about self-respect and feeling worthy of love. I wasn't talking to Kelsey each morning about life and its meaning over a mocha latte and cheese Danish.

The blinders kept me focused on the goal, the outcome, but they kept me from seeing what could be. What should be. What needs to happen to find joy—to find belonging—to find *me* again.

Excited—November 2021

Dear Journal,

Heart and soul spewed all over the page. Words, circles, dates, stars, all of it was there.

My life.

My timeline.

My Big Things.

I had no idea that when I drew them out, the ups and downs would become so apparent, and so drastic. My life seemed to move from one extreme to the next, with time being the only thing separating it.

I sure know how to blow shit up.

Yes, I realize that I might look like a fucked-up mess on paper, but there are reasons for my choices and for some of the things that happened. Surely. There must be.

There must be more, these Big Things that harness everything else that carries so much meaning. I'm starting to notice things like themes of avoidant communication, safety and love, and invisibility. I wonder what role those play. I wonder why I haven't ever noticed them before. I wonder a lot of things, but now I'm excited about what comes next.

~Excited

For You (#TheBigThings)

Dear Seeker,

I once heard someone say that time keeps things from happening all at once. It gives us the ability to have perspective, learn, grow, and change. But I, like so many, didn't use time to its full advantage. I went from one event to the next, trying very hard not to look back and not dig too deep into the *why* of it all. I thought that meant I was searching for something, but now I know I was running, choosing to reject the power of slowing down to reflect while still moving ahead.

At twenty-five, standing toe-to-toe with Frank, I had a choice.

In.

Or out.

I chose to go out into the world, chase dreams, bounce from place to place, and search for a feeling. That didn't get me what I wanted, but it did lead me here, writing to you.

Back then I was running from fear—rejection, abandonment, loneliness— I was running so that I wouldn't face rejection and be unloved. I was afraid that if I allowed someone to see the real me, they would deem me unlovable, because I thought I was. I didn't even know it at the time, but that little girl inside of me, the one who never got what she really needed, reminded me of it in covert ways. Encapsulated by fear, she tried to protect me from pain; she told me to do it—to run.

It wasn't until I started going to therapy that I thought about my life differently. And when I did, things made sense. The various patterns I had been playing out without taking the time to step back and see them were suddenly *very* visible. Like why I kept trusting the same type of man and why they kept letting me down; why I felt so uncomfortable telling Maime I loved her even though I felt it so deeply; and why Poppy's death had such a profound impact on me.

If I had to guess, I'd say that the Big Things in your life look a lot like mine. There in our timeline, we all have births, deaths, and metaphorical rebirths. There are beginnings and endings, and there are highs and lows. There are patterns and messages built into every Big Thing, and there are short and long spans of time in between.

I like to call these Big Things, the fence posts that shape our life.

They are what stands out, our "go-to" when someone says, "Tell me about yourself." These are the things that make sense to us and are usually how we define ourselves. There's so much to learn about who we are by understanding them. So after you've spent time Remembering your Inner Child, next you must **Draw It Out**.

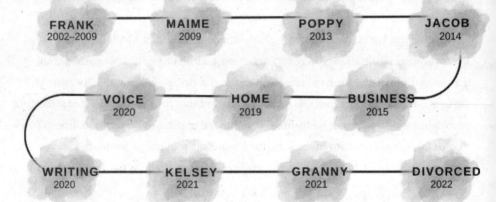

Kasey's Timeline

THE BIG THINGS

FRANK	MAIME	POPPY	JACOB
2002–2009	2009	2013	2014

VOICE	HOME	BUSINESS
2020	2019	2015

WRITING	KELSEY	GRANNY	DIVORCED
2020	2021	2021	2022

Start with a simple horizontal line (or a squiggly one) on a page of your notebook. List the most apparent things, the ones that come right into your memory without much heavy lifting. Like when you graduated high school and moved away, when someone you loved died, or when you got married or had a baby—those are the kinds of things that stick out; those are the Big Things.

Draw a vertical line to notate the year they happened and how you felt. Was it a traumatic (T) experience? The way many therapists define a trauma is anything that exceeds your current coping skills. A trauma overwhelms your central nervous system and pushes you outside your window of tolerance. Regardless of age and demographics, we have all experienced traumas in some capacity.

Note any events where you experienced fear (F)—maybe when your greatest fear came true, maybe when it almost did, or maybe it's something that you still fear. On your timeline, write down significant positive events as well, things that brought you joy (J). Keep drawing it out until you can see the events of your life lying right there in front of you on a page.

Now breathe.

As you draw out how you got to where you are today, I would encourage you not to forget that you are Remembering, not Reliving. You are looking at this timeline of yours from your adult perspective. Reliving is when the past feels as if it is in the now. This does *not* help us make meaning of our lives or help us heal our Inner Child but gets us stuck in the past instead.

If you don't have access to many of these memories, it could be dissociation, which can happen when our brain tries to protect our heart. You can still participate in the exercises, just work with what you can access. You don't have to force it. But above all else, as a Seeker, please don't quit.

Notice years that were particularly hard, and what came before and after. And then, go back into each of those Big Things and look deeper. This exercise caused me to remember my Inner Child in a way that was more vivid and thorough. I was reminded of how at nine years old, eleven, and again at fourteen, I distinctly remember moments when I heard Mom say, "Turn off the music." I remember those words, but how I interpreted them was probably very different from how she remembers. What I heard was: music is noise. Noise is bad. What I understood was that joy was too loud for my mother. So, I suppressed it around her, and eventually, suppressing joy became part of who I was.

I didn't realize how that message and others just like it influenced me and subsequently the Big Things in my life. For the first time, seeing everything out there on paper, I was honest with myself. I wasn't happy. And I had forgotten what joy felt like.

I had somehow landed in a compartmentalized world, one that was focused on moving forward, chasing dreams, and reaching goals—I had a More Mentality, one that kept me searching for the next thing I thought would fulfill me. But no matter what I did, joy never came.

Life is too short not to extract the most meaning we can out of it. As a community of women, of human beings, let's come together, support one another, and look at life through a braver lens. Let's sit down on our red fold-up chair and allow ourselves the space to remember the past, enjoy the present, and dream for our future.

Let's give ourselves a change in perspective; let's sit somewhere different so we can see what it's like for someone else; let's understand our own perspective a little more; and let's open the doors to possibilities. Let's gift ourselves with a front-row seat and watch the making of a new story of our lives unfold before our eyes.

Your Back Porch Bestie,
K

P.S. As I'm sure you can tell, these aren't *all* my Big Things. There are more, and plenty of reasons why I didn't include them. Some are too painful, some too private, and some—well, I'm still processing in therapy. I tell you this because I want you to extend grace to yourself. This doesn't have to be an A+ overachieving school project. This is for you and only you, Seeker. The point is to bring you closer to your true self so that you can experience the joy you deserve.

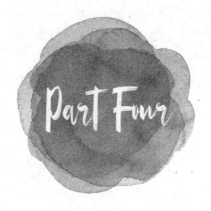

Understanding
THE LITTLE THINGS

• The body remembers. Silenced until an event, a
sound, a sight, a touch, or a word awakens it. •

"I thought I was broken and needed fixing, but
I was actually hurt and needed healing."
~unknown

The Little Things in our lives can be easily overlooked. But when we find the courage to see them, to understand them, we realize that's where meaning lies. Once we open our heart, mind, and body to them, they show themselves and become the connecting fibers of our life.

Auction–January 2022

I didn't see Granny as much as I wanted before she died. I was preoccupied with separating from and ultimately divorcing Jacob, and I was not in the best frame of mind to chitchat about life. I took the kids down to visit her whenever I had the chance, and I spent as many days as possible with her at the hospital before she was moved to the nursing home.

Her house went up for auction fast. No one told me it was happening, and I probably wouldn't have known at all if I hadn't noticed something in her yard one morning on my way to take the kids to school.

With all three in tow, I see a big red and yellow sign beside the road that says, "Absolute Auction, House and Personal Items."

A deep pain explodes from the pit of my stomach, one so deep it hurts all the way up into my chest. I feel it in my arms, in my neck, and even in my eyes. Another trigger. This time for the grief from her death that I haven't fully processed and the knowledge that Pop built this house for her, which stings with finality. I continue driving far enough to pull over into the parking lot of a familiar church.

"Whatcha doin', Mom?" Thayer Bear asks from the back seat.

"Just taking a minute, bud."

Out of the way of traffic, I stare out my windshield, hands trembling, thinking about how many times I watched Granny in her Sunday best hobbling out of this church on her bad knee. I think about how many times I saw Pop wink at one of the church ladies, and how many sticks of chewing gum I got from the deacons that stood right there in the doorway. So many memories are attached to this old Southern Baptist church, this road, and the house built by the men in my family, and to the woman who filled it full of memories.

It was once my escape—my home, the only one I'd truly ever known.

And now what? Now it will be sold to the highest bidder, and I have no say in the matter.

I'd buy it. I want to, but I can't—everything is still tied up in the divorce proceedings. Yet again, another reminder of what little control it feels like I have over my life. All those years I spent with Granny talking about the things she wanted me to have after she was gone means nothing now. The Denim Days figurines that she was so proud of, the cast iron skillets she taught me to sear meat in, and all her hand-me-down coffee cups are going to go to someone who couldn't care less about them. All the things she knew held a special place in my heart—the things she knew I would appreciate when no one else would—I won't get a chance to have them.

———

Starting bid: one dollar.

Are you freaking kidding me?

Kelsey and I sit in the living room one night after dinner. She's been staying with me a lot since August. I feel calmer when she's around. I feel safe talking to her about my feelings, and boy do I have a lot of them now.

Seeing the poorly photographed items from my grandmother's house causes every part of me to want to slam my laptop shut, cuss under my breath, and go on about my life like nothing ever happened—like Granny was still alive. My pain tells me to run. My hurt says to go cry alone in the closet. Don't look, don't feel, don't think, because it hurts too badly. They aren't just things. Some are worth more than the starting bid and some probably aren't, but they are priceless memories of my childhood, the only thing that I have left—the only thing that can help me better understand who I am now.

"Bid on them," Kelsey says.

I debate it, but I do—every single item in the auction, I bid on. Once I start, I can't stop. Thousands of dollars and five truckloads later, I pick up the contents of my Granny's house and take it back to mine.

Crocheted afghans, cement yard ornaments, a set of encyclopedias, and the *National Geographic* magazines I grew up reading over Poppy's shoulder are all right here. The assortment of nonmatching coffee cups, each with a different story that I've heard more than a handful of times, and the red crystal glasses she used to decorate the dining room table for holiday meals are back in my hands where they belong.

I see Pop's cow bells, old wooden pipes, and journals that are meticulously notated with the measurements of how high the water was on Lake Cumberland at different times of the year. I find the brooches Gran wore every Sunday morning and Wednesday evening to church, and the long strand of fake pearls that she liked to wrap around her neck a couple of times before heading out in Black Beauty for a Sunday drive.

Buried deep in the boxes are the raggedy old blankets she used to curl up in her recliner with before bedtime—they still smell like her. Soft, worn, and raggedy—there isn't much left of them, except her memory. Underneath the old phone book, pens, and the desk organizer, I find Poppy's deck of playing cards, in near perfect condition.

My heart smiles.

I touch every single item that once hung on Granny's wall. The one that showcased every celebration, graduation, and birth throughout her lifetime, beginning with her son, Ronnie Gene. In my hands I hold everything that sat on the metal shelves in the bathroom. All the whatnots and doodads strung out all over her house can now be showcased in mine. I look at each thing and spend hours back down on Slate Branch Road, feeling just like I used to, remembering all the Little Things.

Seeker, you're at an important point in the book where my heart and mind are open to Remembering. Because of this, the following stories do not follow a chronological order. They are memories, triggered by objects that I find while going through the remnants of my Granny's life after her passing.

Hang in there, allow yourself to float back into the past with me, linger there amidst my senses, and experience moments for what they are as I'm taken back and forth through Little Things that now actually feel quite big. **Soon, I will ask you to do the same, Seeker.**

Starting to See—March 2022

"Y ou're beginning to understand, aren't you?" my therapist asks six months into therapy.

"Understand what, exactly?"

"The tapestry that's become your life," she says.

I Remember more and more, but the Big Things that show up on my timeline are still hard for me to process. It's tough seeing how everything is so artfully connected. I even feel a bit foolish that I didn't see the connections before now, but that's how it goes. When you're living it, it's hard to see it.

What started as a line with events scattered across my life span has become something so much more. That simple activity has made space for more of my feelings, which have given way to even more memories. Little Things that I never expected to be anything more than tiny, irrelevant details are filling in the gaps and becoming everything.

My awareness of the Big Things has made it possible to understand the importance of the little ones. So I keep going. I write them down as they come to mind— I fill in the gaps of my timeline as I comb through Granny's trinkets and treasures. I've held on to so many memories of my grandparents, hoping to get closer to them with each one, hoping that in some way they will bring me back home.

I spend weeks jotting down things in my quiet moments. Mostly, they come to me in the shower or while I'm driving, and I don't stop them. I don't redirect them. I allow myself to remember it all. Then I add them to my timeline in the spaces where they belong.

Eventually I'll connect them like a thread running through my life, similar to the stitches Granny and I used to make in our throw pillows, uneven and colorful. The Little Things are what I notice.

"Yes," I say finally. "I am beginning to understand."

"How do you feel about that?" she asks.

"I feel."

"Well, that's a good start."

DAUGHTERS

One thing Granny and Lennon had in common was their love of snow globes. Rummaging through a new box from the auction, I spot a miniature Statue of Liberty globe among the other knickknacks, and I experience a feeling that I haven't felt in a long time: comfort.

Like Big Granny pointed out in her garden a million years ago, there's no guessing when it comes to where I come from. There's something around the eyes of all the women in my family—even my mom, though she's not a Mitchell—that speaks kinship.

I've given it a lot of labels over the years—grit, determination, worry lines, love lines—but none of those fully encompass it. It's just something about my family.

I see it now even when I look at my daughters. Lennon and Maime hate to be told they look alike. They hate it even more when someone says they look like me. It pains me to tell you this, girls, but it's true. You are my minis, obvious to anyone with eyes.

It's funny because I didn't realize I was doing it until I had my son, but I raised them to be just like me, too.

Things my mom, Big Granny, and Granny Lillie did with me, for me, I do with and for them. At the time I thought it was harsh, unnecessary, uncomfortable, but now, I know these are the things that turned me into a strong, capable, and confident woman.

"I ain't doin' nary bit for you, that you can do for you'ins own self," Granny would say.

And she didn't. As easy as it would have been for her to intervene, she'd stand to my side, watching, coaching, as I needed it, all to teach me how to be an independent woman.

I understand now that raising daughters requires so much more of me. Living in a world where everything and everyone tries to pull them down and make them question their worth, I need my daughters to be strong, but not too strong.

That's where it gets tricky. It's my job to put them in situations to grow, test themselves, and find their confidence so that later in life they know that they can do hard things. So they can stand up for themselves, ask for what they need, and be fulfilled.

Intentionally or not, the women in my life did this for me, and I will do this for my girls, too. Just as the old snow globes that Granny bought Lennon are to them, my girls are sometimes as perplexing and full of wonder to me. Beautiful and unique, strong but fragile, never knowing what you're going to get with each turn—this is what makes them so much fun, so unpredictable, so uniquely loveable.

SONS

There aren't many photos left from Granny's estate. Dad says most of them are stored away, but some days, I get lucky and find one. Today is that day. It is all too familiar; in fact, I've seen it many times. I always thought Dad looked like the older brother, Wally, on the old TV show *Leave It to Beaver*. Holding the picture of him as a mischievous young man, right before he left for the service back in the fifties, I see myself.

———

More than anything, Granny loved being a mom. Don't get me wrong, I think she loved being a Granny, too, but nothing compared to her Ronnie Gene.

If I heard it once, I heard it a hundred times: she wanted a big family and a house full of kids, but the good Lord only blessed her with one—my dad.

He did no wrong, at least not in her eyes.

She treated all the men in the family differently than the girls. She'd oscillate from favoring my dad, to my brother, then sometimes to Frank when we were together, then to Jacob when I was with him. There is something about being a man that the women in my family tended to favor.

When my son, Thayer, was born, it was as if another blessing had shown up in the cabbage patch garden of Gran's. She worshiped the ground he walked on, but Pop never got to meet him—he was born five years after Pop died. Sometimes I think about what that relationship would have looked like, what nickname he would have picked for Thayer, and what outdoor lesson he'd teach him.

I'm guilty of that same different kind of love for Thayer. And now that I have it, I can see it for what it is. It's not favoritism like I previously thought Granny gave the boys, just different.

Thayer is easy in ways my girls are not. I don't have to worry about making him as strong because I know the world will be kinder to him. In fact, I want him to be soft in all the ways I was raised not to be—open, honest, vulnerable, and emotionally accessible. I want him to be kind and gentle and to love with his whole heart without shame. The world needs more men like that. I want my son to be one of those men.

He's a rambunctious three-year-old, and I love that he's already able to express his emotions better than most of the grown men that I know.

"Mommy, I is just so angry," he says.

"Do you need a minute to calm down?" I ask.

"Yesth," he responds, with the cutest little lisp that makes my heart weak.

That, Seeker, is joy. And that's something I would have missed if I hadn't started on this journey. It makes me think of all the little moments with my kids and wonder how many my parents missed with me.

Two Christmases ago I surprised my dad with a new refrigerator. He didn't expect it and was in total shock when the delivery guys hauled it in through his old front door. I was standing at an angle, but I think I saw a tear in his eye. I'm not sure if it was gratitude, or all the bourbon I'd fed him during dinner, but that night he was emotional in a way I'd never seen from him before.

I read him a chapter in the book I am working on, about him and Poppy "drawing out the day" after their morning coffee. When I finish and look up to meet his eyes, they are cloudy just like mine. I can see him fighting hard with all his might to hide the tears, to keep them deep within the wells of his eyes for no one to see. But I see them.

"You're incredible," he whispers, his voice thick, in a way I'd only heard a couple of times during my childhood. If I wasn't looking straight at him, I might not have even heard him—he is that quiet.

I go on reading, acting as if things are normal, but they aren't. In my head I am saying everything except for the words on the page. This is the first time he has ever been sentimental with me.

My family doesn't hand out compliments, and I realize that night that I don't know how to accept them. Instead, I do the only thing I know to do: I change the subject. But I feel his words and his love, immensely. I feel like, from him anyway, I have finally been given the one thing I've been waiting for my entire life—to be seen, to be appreciated, to be told I am loved by my Old Man.

"How did you feel when your dad said that?" my therapist asks.

"Proud."

It is easier to describe my feelings now. "Fine" doesn't come up as much in conversation as it used to. And I do feel proud. That's what I've always wanted, that's what I think all kids want: for their parents to be proud of them.

For Dad to speak those words must have taken courage. The act alone is everything he has never been. There was no avoidance in that statement, no conflict, no bickering, no use of grand gestures, no searching for helmets, just straightforward communication between a father and a daughter.

"Tell me more."

"I felt like he saw me, all my hard work, the sacrifice, the grit, the determination, pride, perseverance—all of it. It felt like he saw it all and was proud that the woman standing in front of him, the one he used to call Little'n—she did all these things."

I needed to hear those words. I needed to be seen, and I was.

"You felt loved by your dad, didn't you?"

"Yes. I felt loved."

FEET

It's so strange and frightening how your life becomes so public after you're gone. I thought I knew my Granny, but sitting here surrounded by all her things, I feel a little guilty—like I am digging into something that was never meant for me to see.

I've seen Granny's stockings since I was a little girl working with her out in the garden. They aren't anything she'd be ashamed of, but here, holding them in my hands, it feels wrong.

———

Maime was the first great-grandchild born into the family. Poppy couldn't get enough of her little bare feet running around the house, but he didn't quite know what to do with her at the same time. None of the men did. They took her in small doses, running off to smoke, mow the yard, or tend to the fallen tree limbs anytime she started to cry or get a little whiny. Granny was the one who entertained her. She let her color on her dining room floor with markers and didn't mind when they crept off the page and onto the tile.

It wasn't anything out of the ordinary for Maime to become more interested in the crookedness of Granny's toes than in the colors on the page.

"Why you wearin' these, Gwanny?" she asks.

"Those are my pantyhose, darlin', so my feet don't get dirty."

"Why do your toes look like that, Gwanny?"

"Because I'm old, honey."

Maime runs her tiny fingers across Granny's feet, tracing the outline of her crooked toes carefully. Round and around she moves, looking up at Granny every so often to see her reaction. Sitting in the recliner watching them, I think to myself, *I bet Maime is the only person I know who would touch Granny's feet.*

It's funny how we develop aversions to things like feet as we grow up, and as kids we don't think a thing about it. The closest I would have come to touching Granny's feet were those stockings I hold in my hand after she is gone, but as a little girl, Maime didn't mind.

"What is it about feet that troubles you?" my therapist asks.

"I don't know. I guess it goes back to vulnerability and safety," I say.

I remember believing that showing your toes was a risqué thing. I don't remember ever being told that, but it had to have come from somewhere, probably the church I grew up in. It wasn't polite to wear open-toed shoes on Sunday, shirts with spaghetti straps, or shorts that didn't come past your fingertips.

My family didn't talk about sex or anything that might lead to it, but I got an earful from Gran about modesty. Showing off anything the good Lord had blessed you with was frowned upon, and the devil himself must be grinning if a boy looked twice.

The experiences I had growing up in church, listening to Pop and Gran talk about church, and forming my own opinion about church over the years caused me to believe that my body was somehow a sinful thing, as opposed to something to be proud of and comfortable in.

It impacted intimacy in my marriages, which, thinking about it now, I realize I never really had. I never truly felt okay in that way. It felt dirty to express my physical wants or needs, so most of the time I didn't. It seemed wrong to explore my body or accept it for what it is. It felt wrong to let someone so close to me in that way. So I didn't.

My friends call me "backward"—I prefer "old fashioned"—for not joining in on their conversations about men in the bedroom. So when a talk came up several years before this journey started about women in the bedroom, I really didn't know how to react. It was with a large group of people, Kelsey included, in a hot tub in Gatlinburg, Tennessee. It was there that I had my first vulnerable experience and unleashed the tiniest bit of hidden curiosity when sex was brought up. That was the first time I ever felt brave enough to ask a question that had been on my mind ever since I met Kelsey.

"How do two women have sex, anyway?" I asked.

They thought I was joking, so they didn't give me a straight answer. But that didn't stop me from wondering. It also didn't stop me from feeling guilty for wondering.

But our bodies, their functions, and what they are designed to do *should* be talked about. We should release the shame and guilt, and speak what's on our mind, whether it be questions, or curiosities, or to teach our daughters that it's okay to have these questions. I don't want to pass weird, backward ideas on to my children. I want them to see me as someone who is open-minded and open-hearted when it comes to sensitive topics.

I never want them to think how they look or who they love is wrong. Something as insignificant as toes should never make them feel uncomfortable or out of place.

CHRISTMAS DO-OVER

Ever since I was old enough to bicker, I teased Granny about her Christmas placemats that I hold in my hands now. Solid berry red shreds of fabric with white lace stained from years of hungry hands that she made all by her lonesome.

I walk in for the first day of holiday break at eighteen years old to see something new spread out across the table. She's made new ones. She watches me carefully as I storm in and pick one up, tracing the stiches carefully with my pointer finger.

"Does it suit you?" she asks.

"Suits me just fine," I say with a smile.

She is happy someone noticed. I always do.

———

I think back to when I was married to Jacob; Lennon is little, and we are renting a nice two-story house in a family-focused subdivision. This is a nice upgrade from where we lived while I was pregnant with her. It is a little more than we can afford, but I am hopeful that the extra strain on my pocketbook will motivate me to make it work. I tell myself that re-creating traditions with my own kids will help me feel better about losing Pop. I want traditions to feel as special to them as they did to me.

Finally, we have a place that is large enough and nice enough that we can invite people over. In fact, the first thing I thought of when I looked at the house was that it would be a perfect place to host Christmas breakfast, and our kids can have a memory like I used to have.

My business is new, and we still don't have much, but things are getting better, and we are recovering from the bankruptcy as well as expected. I worked all year to save enough money to buy a decent Christmas tree with real ornaments, not just the ones the kids made and brought home from school, so I decorate the house as festively as I can. I give it my all, creating something that resembles what Granny used to create for me.

It is not much, but it does feel homey. The kids like it. We invite his family to do Christmas at our house this year, and we are all so excited. *I* am so excited— finally a chance to make up for lost traditions and time. I plan for weeks, making sure everything is up to par. I research the recipes that I used to love growing up, and I plan for each and every person to have a thoughtful gift.

Christmas comes quickly, but his family doesn't. Something comes up at the last minute and they decide to do the holidays at someone else's house instead. I am heartbroken. It hurts me badly, and I feel like I am not worthy of such an important holiday tradition. It feels personal, so I push them away in my heart. I build walls to protect myself. I lower my expectations of what a family should be so that I won't be disappointed again.

I just want someone to notice me, my effort, my contribution, and my love.

———

A history of abandonment trauma will lead you to inadvertently sabotage your relationships to affirm your fears, because, after all, they are what we keep close.

During Christmas 2016, I wasn't thinking about that. I was thinking about how hurt and angry I was with Jacob and his family. How that was a trigger for me, taking me back to feeling hurt by my own family. In those moments I didn't understand my own pain, so I didn't know what to do with it. I withdrew even further from people and situations that could hurt and disappoint me again.

Unhealthy attachments to parental figures in childhood can also lead to taking happenstance situations personally in adulthood. It leads to putting up more walls to protect the remaining pieces of a broken heart.

Conversation and conflict weren't things Jacob or our families knew how to handle—he didn't have much more experience with healthy relationships than I did. We only knew how to avoid things. So each and every time we had a fight, we buried our hurt down a little deeper and pretended we were fine. We thought that if we pretended hard enough it would become true, but it never did.

I made myself believe that this change of holiday plans was just a Little Thing—that he didn't notice how much creating those memories with our family meant to me, and that was okay. He didn't see what I saw—that my family was withering away like the leaves of Pop's maple trees. I probably should have realized that this was a clear symptom of a much larger problem, but I didn't.

The hurt just festered down there below the surface. It lay there ignored and rotting, only to turn into a poison that caused me to be triggered by sounds, smells, and virtually anything that pokes an unhealed wound. The hurt compounds and becomes so toxic that it spills over into all facets of life until we acknowledge that it's there and commit to healing it.

PAJAMAS

Another weekend spent going through Granny's belongings, and I find a nightgown of all things—high neck, lace collar, long sleeves with ruffled elastic wristbands.

Sexy, Granny. Sexxxxyyyyyy.

If anyone was going to end up with it, I guess I'm glad it's me. I bet she's looking down right now, wiping her brow with relief that it didn't land in some old goat's auction winnings. Pop sitting beside her, shaking his head, embarrassed as usual.

"I'll get Thayer a bath and get him ready for bed," Kelsey says to me after I come home late from a stressful meeting with my attorney. "Just go lie down."

I need to rest—mentally, physically, emotionally, all of it. I need a break but that is not an option, so I take her up on her offer. She's been staying with me more and more these days, and the kids seem to be happy that there's another person here to give them attention. They've known her as long as I have because of their run-ins with one another at the office, and they enjoy her being around.

I lie there and stare up at the ceiling, thinking about the holidays that are right around the corner, particularly about how this year will look a lot different for my kids.

"Hey, Kase, where are Thayer's pajamas?" Kelsey hollers from his room, upstairs.

I sit straight up in bed as if a bolt of thunder sounded outside my window.

"Umm. He doesn't have pajamas."

My kid doesn't have pajamas. Why did I stop buying him pajamas?

"Everything changed when *I* stopped getting pajamas on Christmas Eve," I say.

"What changed?" my therapist asks.

Every year, even when I became an adult, Granny bought all the grandkids pajamas to open on Christmas Eve. The next morning, we ate breakfast wearing them and opened our presents still dressed in them, and it wasn't until we took them off that evening that we knew the holiday was over.

When Pop died in 2013, so did that tradition, and it wasn't until I saw Granny's nightgown that I remembered and made the connection. They were gone just like he was, so I blocked that memory from my mind. It was still there, though; I just buried it deep. If I am being honest with myself, I blame Granny, and I spent years doing my best to avoid everything that reminded me of what I lost. I no longer touched the traditions I once looked forward to the most. Instead, I opted to try on new ones, like trying on a sweater, hoping to find something that would fit, that would make the holidays feel warm and safe again. But despite every effort, they never did.

"So what changed?" she asks.

"I guess we all did."

CLOSETS

Granny kept all her most prized possessions stacked in the bottom of her and Poppy's closet. When she started to get sick, I'd pull a few things out every time I went down there to visit. She spent her life putting photo albums together, writing little notes in the margins, and listing the date they were taken and the ages of each person in them. I snuck out one here and there and hung it in my office.

After a few months' worth of visits, I gathered pictures of her and the Old Man walking across Natural Bridge when he was about the same age as my little boy, Poppy's driver's license from the 1980s, Granny's grade school report card with a note from her teacher about how she talks too much, and some of Poppy's old stone Mason pins of which he was so proud.

Now, the vintage baby hangers I hold in my hands take me right back to a memory that happened just a few weeks ago.

———

"What are you doing?" Kelsey asks.

I can't answer her. Down on my knees, in the farthest corner from the door, I raise my head enough to catch a glimpse of myself in the floor-to-ceiling mirror. I see her instead.

"Why are you in here?" she asks.

I try to turn and look at her, but my eyes are filled with too many mascara-stained tears—I can only see the outline of her body. I look down and watch the black droplets freckle the carpet. I sense her approaching me from behind, then she bends down and puts her arms tightly around me.

I have been in the closet crying for a while. I'm not sure of the time; she's here after work, and this started after lunchtime when I got an unexpected text from my attorney. She doesn't yet know that all my emotions are coming to a head. My body feels dysregulated, my feelings are all over the place, and I can't help but wonder if "the change" is about to happen. One minute I'm confident, the next minute I only think the worst.

Despite the work I'm doing on myself, in moments like these, I feel like such a failure. I've been putting on a good front since filing for divorce. I certainly don't want to add any more stress to her than necessary.

With my head leaning back against her chest, she says, "Talk to me." When I relax into her, she turns me around so she can look me in the face. I wriggle down so it's harder for her to see me. I feel the deep wrinkles between my eyes and forehead, the tears, and the snot. It's all I imagine she sees in this moment.

Instead, she is patient and warm. Her compassion for me goes deep; she sees beyond my mess of a face into my heart. She is concerned about my pain and nothing else.

I can't muster up the words to explain my feelings, so she tells me to cry instead.

"Let it out. It's going to be okay."

"What was your experience with crying like before this?" my therapist asks.

Someone following me around trying to fix whatever was wrong with me, assuming it was about them. Someone who'd become so defensive that an argument was sure to happen, one where I'd need to defend myself against my own feelings.

"Different," I say. "No one has ever told me to let it out. No one has ever told me it was okay to cry."

"What did they say instead?"

I can't remember the words exactly, but I remember the feeling. Shame. Embarrassment. Weakness.

"When my mom and dad finally divorced, my mom remarried a man, and they built a little A-frame cabin forty-five minutes outside of town. My bedroom was the only room in the upstairs loft."

"The one where you peed off the roof?" she asks.

"Yep. There were two closets, two half triangles that were long and narrow, and that's where I stayed most of the time when they were home."

They weren't tall enough for me to stand up in, but they were plenty long enough for a pillow, blanket, and my see-through landline phone.

"I spent most of my time in that closet," I tell her.

"Why?"

"Well, I didn't have a cell phone back then, and since the house was small and open, with a spiral staircase connecting the basement to my bedroom, my mom and stepdad could hear everything I said and did, so I stayed in the closet to keep quiet."

I stretched the cord to my phone all the way through the center of the room so that it would be quietly tucked away. I turned the ringer off, where it only lit up when it rang, not to disturb anyone. Mom even set me up with my own phone line so that if my friends called, it wouldn't ring to the whole house, just my closet.

"What was that like for you?"

"Safe in my closet."

Ahh. I have been looking for safety. Of course.

"What about someone telling you it's okay to cry?" she asks.

"Weird."

Crying has never felt safe, which makes sense as to why I tried to do it in secret—why I never shared that side of me with anyone. Because it wasn't safe.

"But it was the closest thing to love that I've ever felt."

TEARS

I stumble across a picture of Poppy holding a crying baby Maime when she was about a year old. This was rare, especially for someone to catch on camera. Normally, at the first sound of a squeal, he'd sit her down and run out the garage door for a secret smoke.

He sure loved her, though, and you could tell how proud he was of her in the picture, tears and all.

———

When I see Lennon enter the room with crocodile tears, my chest tightens, my shoulders grow knots, and I breathe through my nostrils, but I disguise my tension.

"What's the matter?" I ask.

"Maime wouldn't get me ice cream," she says.

She's not too happy when she doesn't get her way.

"Why's that so upsetting to you?" I ask.

More tears. Now, gasping to breathe, she spits water from her eyes and snot from her nose, which lands in the center of my face.

"Lennon!" I say, annoyed. "I said, what's wrong?"

"I don't know."

"If you're going to cry and not tell me what's wrong, then go to your room."

As she turns to run toward her room, I stop everything. Breathing, speaking, moving—I realize what I have just done.

———

I used to tease my employees about crying, who later adopted my saying, *Go cry in the car.* I never knew where that little thought came from, but I do now. Until I reconnected with my Inner Child and was taken back to my mom's tearstained Cutlass and all the feelings that happened there, I didn't realize where my emotional intolerance came from.

It is how I was programmed.

I was taught not to cry, and if I did, I needed to do it where no one could see or hear me. When Lennon cried and couldn't tell me what it was that I could fix, it triggered me, and I went right back to when I remembered all the tears I had shed alone in my closet. I remembered why I believed I couldn't let anyone see me, and why I needed to hide my vulnerability. I remembered why I felt safe in the closet. All I needed was someone to tell me it was okay to cry.

I never did that to Lennon again. I look back and realize how differently I might have felt if I was given the permission to let it out as a kid. My family's own lack of emotional intelligence was like a dam holding back water; the amount of pressure and eventual pain that put on my little heart could have all been released if I had known it was okay to let it out.

Now, I let Lennon see me cry. I talk about how I feel. I ask her how she feels. I'm curious about her emotions. Now, she comes to me with a feeling, and I help her understand it. Because now, I know that until we understand, change can never happen.

PATRIARCHY

I'm not sure why, but as I sit here going through dishes, cigars, and cattle bells, for Christ's sake, something keeps cycling through my mind. I hear the words, over and over like a chant, and all I can do is feel the remnants—the leftover emotions, tethered to a past that I don't yet fully understand.

Protect the man.

Protect the man.

Protect the man.

"Kels, I need to ask you something," I say. Without waiting for an acknowledgment, I continue. "I see my grandpa's things, which makes me think about, not just him, but the men in my life, past and present. My dad, my brother, uncles, all of them."

She's fiddling with something, but she stops and looks at me when I say the word *men*.

When I go through Granny's things, "I hear, 'protect the man,' in my head over and over," I say. "Why do you think that is?"

I've never had conversations like these. Is it because I've only ever attempted it in a relationship with a man? Is it because women look at things differently—internalize things differently? Neither Frank nor Jacob would have understood the question I am asking her.

"I understand what you're saying, and I think I know why," she says.

In a family of strong women, there are Little Things that indicate that "we," even me, always protect the man, no matter what.

The women in my family are known to start their husband's car in the morning so they don't get cold. They shield them from the stressors of their children. They do everything they can to meet their needs before they ever have to ask. The women will work three jobs so the man doesn't have to work overtime at one. They tell the children the sugar-coated version of things so they don't have to hear the honest truth about their father. Any way you look at it, women protect men.

But why?

Why now, after everything, after all the hurt, all the betrayal, all the loss, do I still feel compelled to make sure the men in my life, past and present, are okay? Why the hell do I do that? And why doesn't it piss me off more than it does? Why do I carry around their burdens so that my children don't have to know that a man is weak? Why do I wear the weight of the responsibility like a backpack that I refuse to put down or return to its rightful owner?

Why?

Why do "we," as women, as a family, overlook the lies, the manipulation, and the greed to protect the ones who vowed to protect *us*?

Why?

Why protect the man when we deserve to be protected, too?

Why are they praised for spending a little time with their own children, and the first second a woman chooses to care for herself, she is cast out, shamed, and judged for thinking about herself for a change. Why do they get the benefit of the doubt, why are they considered the underdogs, when we are the ones who sacrifice and fight for the one thing that no one ever gives us credit for—*BEING A WOMAN.*

It's hard. The prerequisite is strength. The way we become strong is through exercise—those murky waters, even. Putting one foot in front of another when what lies ahead is not going to let up. Knowing that we have to keep moving, not because it will get easier, but because we have to. We have people who depend on us, need us, because we're women.

This is what we do.

"Why do we accept it?" I ask. "This idea of being a superwoman, of being everything to everyone in our lives?"

"Because we're supposed to."

I want to challenge her, but she *is* right. Is it because we don't understand where it comes from, or because we're doing what we were told to do? Is it because we are perpetuating a cycle of intergenerational trauma, and, unbeknownst to us, we are the only ones who can stop it?

"That doesn't sit well with me," I say.

"Then do something to change it."

SUITCASES

In the corner of my garage, I see a set of suitcases: big, medium, and small. All three a faded collegiate blue, but, nonetheless, they appear to be in good condition.

I almost didn't bid on the set, but at the last second, I did. I don't remember much about them because I never in my life saw Poppy or Granny use one. I never knew them to travel or stray far from home. These three suitcases were neatly stowed in the coat closet as soon as you entered their front door. They were there, probably from before I was born, and they remained there until December 2021 when Granny died.

It takes all my might to swallow the lump in my throat when I see her walking down the stairs holding a suitcase.

"Where are you going?" I ask.

She doesn't hear me.

Life is crazy right now. We are both trying to create a new normal, navigate through two divorces, and figure out how to communicate with one another. I am making progress on a personal note—therapy is helping, but I still have a lot of things to unlearn.

She doesn't want me anymore.

I'm not enough for her either.

It's all just too much to handle.

I begin to cry.

She looks up, and we make eye contact. Her forehead crinkles, and she sets the suitcase down.

"What's wrong?" Kelsey says.

"You're leaving."

"No, honey. I'm just bringing this suitcase downstairs to pack for our trip."

A sigh of relief engulfs my body. I'm flooded with emotion, both relief and embarrassment.

"You're triggered by a suitcase, aren't you?" she asks.

"I think so. I had no idea."

Each time Frank and I got into a serious argument I responded by telling him I wanted a divorce. I didn't, but if anyone was going to leave, it was going to be me. I needed to beat him to the punch. It would hurt too badly for him to leave me.

Each time Jacob and I got into an argument, he left. And left. And left again, carrying a suitcase.

Over time, I learned that conversations are not solutions, but leaving is. When things get too hard, you leave. When things become unbearable, you leave. This is wrong, and I know that now, but only until I started trying to understand myself did I see it.

The Little Things are everything.

———

Mom said Dad used to leave.

Mom said we used to leave.

Mom said Poppy used to leave.

My childhood was full of leaving.

My adulthood is full of leaving.

It is dysfunctional.

It is not a solution to conflict.

It doesn't feel good.

I don't want to leave any more.

ACCESS POINT 26

When I was about the same age as Lennon, my Granny and I spent one Saturday in summer on a beach-inspired art project. As I hold it in my hands some thirty years later, I'm in awe that she was able to keep it safe this long.

Outside on the metal patio furniture, she hands me a mason jar, some cement mix, and a bag of seashells that she says she brought back from the ocean. I believe her. I have no reason not to.

We take our time lathering the cement onto the jar and plop the seashells on it while it is still wet. We each make our own and talk the entire time.

"What are you going to do with your jar?" she asks.

"Don't know yet. Probably put my paintbrushes in there."

"I might do that, too," she says.

She is so curious. She wants to know how I think, what my favorite color is, and how I like my eggs cooked. She wants to know what size pants I wear and if I've grown out of my training bra yet. She asks me how I feel about things, and how I think she should decorate the living room.

Until the moment I hold the jar in my hands again, I haven't thought another thing about that day out on the porch. But now I do. Now it's a symbol of hope, love, and family. I have no idea what she did with it back then—whether she put paintbrushes in it or not, but she kept it safe for me. But now, here in my hands, with a few missing seashells, the memories of her are stronger than ever.

———

With a book on my lap and the sun beaming down on my shoulders just off Access Point 26, a straw hat perched on my head, I can close my eyes and relax for the first time in months.

Fripp Island is beautiful in the fall. The beach is peaceful around Access Point 26, the water is warm, and the shrimp boats are always coming in from a big run.

I am still going to therapy, and I'm focused on understanding all that I have remembered so far. It is not the first time I've been here in this spot on the beach, but to my body, it feels like it.

The water is dark blue, the sand is hot, and the fighter jets from Parris Island fly low. The Bonito Boathouse is still there by the dock, the turkey and mayo sandwiches from the deli taste the same, and I take the same route every evening to watch the sunset over the abandoned house on Pritchard's Island.

All familiar, all the same.

It's interesting how our primal body seeks out the familiar. Perhaps that's how we so easily revert to old habits, same types of people, and the same problems.

The seashells are small, much like the ones on the mason jar I made with Granny. Every night when the sun goes down, I eat the same butter pecan ice cream—Poppy's favorite. There's comfort in the predictability. I buy bags of ice from the same ship store and creep up ever so sneakily on the same pond hoping to get a glimpse of Sherman.

All familiar, all still the same.

The beach house I bought a year ago during the COVID-19 pandemic looks the same. The last time I was here was with Maime for AJ's editing retreat. It has the same beachy cottage smell that it did the first time I looked at it with my realtor. I take a shower in the same bathroom with the green tile to rinse off the day, just like I always do.

Lennon and Thayer are here with me, and they love this island just as much as I do. Kelsey is here with me this time, too; that is different. Last time, I sat in this same spot on the beach and listened to a song that made me think of her, but I never told her—I didn't tell anyone.

My favorite spot on the island is no different than it ever was. A tiny white crab scurries across the tips of my toes, running toward a hole that he likely calls home. Little things like this is why my kids like it here so much. I smile when I see his beady eyes. I do more than smile. I laugh. I laugh out loud.

I look far out into the water, searching for the line where the sky meets the ocean, and breathe the saltwater deep into my body—hoping it will cleanse me, heal me from whatever still holds me back. I swallow the air in until my head feels fuzzy, then let it out slowly. I melt into my chair, feel the coolness of the waves tickle my feet, and wonder if Kelsey notices the freckles on my legs.

I am happy.

Completely present in the moment, free from the judgment of others, free from the responsibilities of life, I am starting to feel alive again. There's hope in my heart that the chaos still lingering from when I chose to leave Jacob will soon turn to peace. I release all the doubt brewing inside me and accept the possibility of any outcome instead.

Will my mom accept this new relationship? How will this choice impact my business? And what will my friends think of me now?

There's still some internal struggle, although I know it's too late to change my mind about him, and about her—I know any other choice than the one I am making wouldn't be the right one.

So many times I sat on this beach, watching these waves, with feelings buried as deep down as I could get them. But this time, I don't do that. I don't bury fears or feelings; I let them go instead. I release them into the saltwater air, out into the ocean, wherever they want to go, because they belong somewhere other than inside of me now.

TIGER EYES

Granny had the most random things. I can't help but wonder how she ended up with it all. I never once knew someone to buy her a decorative hawk, which she found to be most appropriate as a living room decoration, perched high on one of the living room trusses. I never once saw anyone gift her with a stuffed dog with roller skates, but nevertheless, she had one.

In the far back bedroom of her house, in the room that she called "hers," lay a tiger. Nearly as large as the smallest grandchild, it was white and had piercing green eyes. Each time the kids visited Granny, they wanted to go back to "her" room and take a ride on the tiger.

She always indulged them, so I'd play along. Now, over in the corner of the garage that we've finally cleared out, bright-eyed Lennon, upon returning from the beach, has the chance to lay claim to it.

———

It feels good to be back home, even if it does mean leaving a place I love. I shower because it's been a long day, and I have a headache. It feels good to let the water roll down my back and let my thoughts and feelings flow.

I have two little blond girls in my bed watching YouTube, and Kelsey lies beside them filling out a timesheet for work. Before I get up and grab a pair of underwear and a tank top to change into, I notice her left arm and the tiger tattoo staring me. She got it soon after we started seeing each other. She says it's *my* green eyes on its face, but I pretend I don't believe her. I catch a quick glimpse of the light from the computer on her face.

You're beautiful.

Water beats down on my neck that hurts so bad from the sunburn. Rapid-fire thoughts come into my mind. Thoughts about therapy, about love, about kids. Do I want more, or do I have enough?

I'd love to have one that's ours.

Men. I can't even picture myself with a man again. *Is that weird?*

Does this mean I'm gay?

Marriage. How do I ask a woman to marry me? And should I?

As I listen to music, feeling it in my heart, I also feel her out there—I feel her with me all the time now. Everywhere I go, she's there with me. I ask myself whether that's normal, but then realize I don't know what normal is anymore—I've come to expect that my normal is different from everyone else's, and for the first time in my life, I accept it.

I think about our story and how I will bring it to the end here in this book, and I realize I don't want it to end, ever. I think back about an hour prior when she walked into my bedroom. I sat in the dark in a sports bra and high-waisted pants. Half my hair was in a high ponytail like a Shih Tzu puppy, and the other half fell over my shoulders. The computer was on my lap, and I was writing about her, but she didn't know that. I caught her looking at me, shaking her head ever so slightly. I felt her looking, but I kept writing. She moved slowly into the bathroom, and a few minutes later, I felt it again. Those eyes on me just like they were at the book launch. I looked over my left shoulder, and there she was, standing in the darkness, where I wouldn't notice, watching me write.

It feels different. She always watches me in a certain way; I don't feel the need to prove anything, other than how much I love her. I don't need to show her that I am right and she is wrong. I don't need her to regret the way she treats me to teach her a lesson. She's not a cookie baking in the oven that I hover over, anxiously watching to make sure it turns out right.

She watches me because she loves me, and I let her because I love her, too. For the first time in my life, it feels good allowing someone to look without having to tell them to, whether it is spoken aloud or just a thought inside my head. It feels good that someone wants to because I make them want to get to know me better.

As she stands in the darkness of my closet doorway, I know what she is thinking because I am thinking the same thing.

It's *you.*

Eight—April 2022

We've talked a lot about feelings, and how important it is to express them to those in your life. "Let's go back to our rating scale for a minute, if that is okay," my therapist says. "How assertive have you been with your feelings over the last couple of weeks?"

I told someone exactly how I felt when they hurt my feelings a few days ago. I also had a run-in with a former employee, a homophobic hypocrite, and I was nice to him. Not because I was fake, but because I had forgiven him for what he said about me, and I genuinely didn't have any negative feelings. I'd met up with an old high school friend for dinner and drinks, and I allowed myself to be vulnerable. I had a deep conversation with him about his feelings and mine, and how our lives turned out twenty years after graduation.

"I'd say a solid eight," I tell her.

"Okay, great. One more question: How much would you say you've loved yourself over the last couple of weeks?"

I remember this question from our first conversation months ago. I didn't know what that meant then, but now I'm starting to. In just the last two weeks, I've seen Jacob's new girlfriend vacationing with him at the beach house I worked so hard to buy, and I felt okay about it. I didn't compare myself, question my worth, or ask for pity publicly. I know I'm worthy of more, and I stand strong. When I needed it, I took time for myself without feeling guilty about it.

"Another eight," I tell her.

"Okay, let's get started. Has anything come up this week that you want to focus on?"

"The book that I'm working on is starting to take shape. Right now, a lot has come up for me about joy. I think that's what's been missing from my life."

I talk about the music, the concerts, the water, and the alone time. As a child, joy was found in the trees, at the sewing machine, and coming from the vinyl record player in the living room at my grandparents' house. I was wild and free and supported in whatever it was I wanted to be. I can't recall joy at Mom's apartment or Dad's trailer, but it was there in the house with the Granny wall. It was hopping on the back of Frank's motorcycle, holding on with all my might. It was anticipating the wheelie as we crossed the bridge on the Cumberland Park-way in the middle of the night. It was there when I didn't yet know how cruel the world could be, when I was still naïve and hopeful, before I ever had anyone make me doubt my self-worth. Joy was there when the moment I was in was all there was.

I recognized it in my body, the twinges of life that flowed through me. Now I look back at old photos and recognize it in my smile. I see it in the innocence of my eyes. Playing sports in high school, sitting in my Poppy's lap at Christmas, and traveling to new places; it was there. It was there back then, but I lost it. Now I'm starting to wonder if maybe it wasn't lost after all. Maybe I shut it down. Could it be that all the Little Things made more of an impact on me than I thought? Maybe I fought against it so hard because I didn't think I was worthy, and I forgot where to find it.

"It sounds like joy has always been found in the refuge from your day-to-day life," she says. "Back then, it revolved around your grandparents' house, and now, it seems like it's being anywhere but home."

Oh shit. Why did I, why do I need to escape to be happy?

I transform into my nine-year-old self again, making ham salad sandwiches in the food processor, drinking an ice-cold Mr. Pibb from the fridge in the garage, and watching my Granny put lipstick on yard ornaments. There, with them, I could be free. If I wanted to make curtains, we sewed. If I wanted to bake, we made pies. If I wanted to make money, we made crafts and sold them. My dreams were always possible, and the journey was always fun. She is right: Granny and Poppy were my escape; that's where my joy lived.

Joy was always something "out there," not something that lived "in me." Finding it and feeling it meant escaping the daily routine of life. Joy isn't part of the day-to-day. It is separate. It is something that must be found in an environment that is emotionally safe, free of judgment, and full of unconditional love.

"Unknowingly, you carried this concept into your adult life," she says. "You saw joy and life as two separate things, never to be experienced together."

"Because that's all I knew."

With Jacob and the kids, we created the idea that experiencing joy only came from planning moments of escape, and even when they happened, it was still missing. We had to go away, buy concert tickets, get a hotel for the weekend, take the kids on a Disney cruise for a fighting chance at joy.

"You don't need to leave your life to find happiness," she says.

I guess I don't need to be busy to make memories either. All that chasing is merely a distraction from the thing that is getting in my way—fear. Distractions exist so I don't have to settle in and look around at my life—so I don't have to find joy in the day-to-day moments—so I don't have to remember the joy that stopped when the ones I loved died, when I lost my safe place, and when I made the wrong choices.

I look out the window and take a breath before mustering up the courage to speak what I know needs to be said. I wait a long time before I say a word.

"I am sending a message to my kids that happiness isn't found at home, aren't I? I'm telling them that they must go away to find joy. It must be an escape for them like it was for me. I'm laying the same foundation that I had."

I sit quietly, staring out the window until the "session is almost over timer" goes off. So many lessons I must unlearn, so many new ones to discover, and here I am, thirty-seven years old, experiencing life again for the first time. Joy means everything. It means I can experience happiness anywhere, with anyone, to whatever level I desire. It means that joy is up to me and my ability to live in a moment.

I realize my relationship to joy changed early in life, shaped by my immediate family. When my mom told me to turn off the music, she was really saying was that joy was meant to be quiet. When my dad didn't do what he promised, he taught me that joy was dependent on acts of service. When my sister treated my joy like a burden, she taught me to hide my happiness around others. When my brother gave up who he was to seek out approval from the men in his life, he taught me that joy was contingent on what people think about you.

My experiences through the years groomed me to compartmentalize my feelings, to protect the vulnerable ones that are bound to get me hurt. After Frank, my tank was empty, and I was hell-bent on never feeling again. I was scared to ever tap back into that softer side because I knew it could be painful. That's when I put my blinders on and went straight for the safest bet, the one who wouldn't necessarily challenge me emotionally, and the one I thought had too good of a heart to break mine: Jacob.

And it worked. I became successful with minimal feelings involved. My blinders allowed me to focus on my strengths, starting one business that led to several more. Before long I bought my first new car. After that I bought my first home. I increased my net worth strategically, and by thirty-six, I had over seven figures in the bank.

I found confidence in my mistakes, my learning curves, and my strengths. More importantly, for the first time in a long time I felt like I belonged somewhere. I found people who understood and supported me, and I didn't feel alone. I felt like I had something meaningful to contribute to help others. But at the end of the day, despite my success and budding confidence, I went to bed alone, without conversation or connection, and, sadly, without joy. Because I was home, and joy didn't live there.

Since I sat down with pen in hand, big blue notebook on my lap, my life has already started to change. It's getting better. With every memory, every connection, and every emotion, I create more space for joy.

"How's the divorce going?" my therapist asks.

"Um, it's going."

We are getting closer to finalizing the split, and that makes me happy. I'm ready to release more baggage and use what I've learned to make a better life for myself and my kids.

"One day," she says, "when you feel like dating again, you'll be in a better place to give *and* receive love."

Dating again? I look away. I haven't told her about Kelsey. Well, that's not true. She knows about her, just not that we have decided to move in together. My therapist and I have a good therapy rhythm going; we've focused on patterns and realizations; and I'm not ready to derail that progress to talk about this. Plus, I don't even really know what *this* is yet.

"I look forward to that—and Portugal," I say. "But there is something on my mind today." I pause to get my thoughts together. "It's funny how life works. The sense of humor it has. In the moments, all the little moments, it feels so bad. Painful. Confusing. Hard. And it is all those things, but when you zoom out and you give yourself the space to look back on all the Big Things that happened, the Little Things are what stand out."

I started with nothing more than a line, dates, and big events on a page, and now, it's the smell of Granny's coffee that I remember, the color of her lipstick, the ridges of Pop's fingernails. How he kept his ink pen in his shirt pocket and spearmint gum in there, too. Now I can remember how I learned to have patience: from watching Poppy play solitaire. The Little Things taught me that.

"My life isn't perfect, but it isn't full of big traumas, either. It was the little ones, the good and the bad, that shaped my Inner Child and because she's still in there begging for me to notice. I neglected her for quite some time, but boy how she's influenced me."

"Yes, she's speaking to you," she says. "We create protective parts of ourselves when we get hurt. We create something that protects that little girl from feeling abandoned again."

"It protects her from being disappointed, too?"

"Yes. It also protects her from her fears. Those that include being controlled, needing others, and constantly being let down. It does all the things that keep her from getting back into a situation that can harm her again."

I've recognized something happening in my body when someone tries to control me, tells me what to do, questions me, doubts me, follows me, or takes my personal space. I fight. It feels like I'm being smothered. Like I'm claustrophobic, like I have to get out. Like I have to run.

"That's *her* speaking to you because she's wounded. Kasey, that exiled part, that protector, created the grit that you have now."

That was something I needed to help me cope with my feelings.

"You knuckled down, worked hard, built businesses, proved to yourself that you could do it, and you did. And here's the good part," she says. "You did those things so that that little girl would never need to depend on someone who might leave her."

It was a way my Inner Child was trying to protect me; I just never saw it as that.

"But that's not good, right?"

"It's not good, and it's not bad," she says. "It's something that happens to all of us. We must be able to see it, and sometimes we need help with that."

"Jacob told me I needed therapy because I was crazy, but I just needed someone to help me zoom out and see the connections between all the things that happened. After months of coming into my own, I know myself better than I ever have, and I know that I'm not crazy."

"You're not crazy. You're strong." A smile beams across her face. "Why do you think I asked you how much you love yourself in our first session?"

Ahh.

"Because without self-love, I'm not strong enough to face my fears, comb through my past, and remember hard things. I needed that—still do," I say.

Because when I love myself, I don't need to worry about anyone leaving me. Because I am enough. I am worthy of love, *even if* it is only from myself.

"Because when you love yourself, you see the world differently."

Laundry Detergent–December 2022

G ranny liked to tell people she was from "up north."
She wasn't.

One time, when we were mid-bicker about how you pronounce Cincinnati, she told me that if you're from "up yonder you's sound more sophisticated."

I hold her dictionary in my hands, the one she liked to study up on once and a while, while I pilfer through the pages looking for any of her chicken scratch in the margins. I think about Kelsey.

———

It's my second trip to Wisconsin to visit Kelsey's family since we've started dating. I thought my city was small, but nothing I've ever seen compares to this one.

"I don't know how you didn't end up with one of your cousins," I say.

She and her mother simultaneously belt out a laugh. "I did," Kelsey says. "Luckily, Mom told me it was my cousin before anything too freaky happened."

Why am I not surprised?

Being there, watching her surrounded by the people she loves, makes me both happy and so incredibly sad. Happy for her that she has a healthy bond with her mom, but sad that I can't say the same, even though my relationship with mine is getting better.

Six days into the trip, I start to get homesick. I miss my kids. Maime, who's thirteen now, texts me at least forty times, asking when I'll be home. As I sit in the recliner, responding to her texts, Kelsey's mom comes in through the back door and hollers in our direction.

"Got ya some laundry detergent."

"Thanks, Mother."

I note what just happened, then I go back to my phone to answer Maime's next question.

> **Maime:** How would you feel if I married Drake, the rapper?
>
> **Me:** I thought you didn't want to get married.
>
> **Maime:** Well, I would marry him. Or someone that looks like him.

Isn't it funny how history repeats itself? Much like the conversations I initiated with Granny on Sundays, Maime is trying to understand my beliefs, my limits, and the conditions of my love. But unlike Granny, with my kids, there are none.

> **Me:** I don't care who you marry—I don't care if you ever get married—as long as you are happy, that's all that matters!

This is an opportunity for me to parent her differently than I was parented.

"Kels," I say to her as we settle down for bed that night. "Your mom knows that you only use a certain kind of laundry detergent to wash your underwear."

"Of course she does. Why?"

"Mine wouldn't."

I don't think anyone in my family knows much about me. Not my favorite color or food, and certainly not what kind of life I dream of having. They don't know my fears, insecurities, or what keeps me up at night. I don't even think they know what I do for work. Granny was the only one who ever asked me questions like that.

While it's a painful realization, I understand what it means: it means that I need to try harder to get to know my children. Because that's one of the ways they will know they're loved.

Asheville–July 2022

Dear Journal,

Today I went back to one of my favorite places on Earth—Asheville, North Carolina—and I took my new favorite human. She told me there was something she wanted to show me.

Dressed up, walking the streets in Battery Park, we turned a corner and entered heaven. The Book Exchange, where we love to indulge in a charcuterie board and a flight of champagne, was built in the 1920s, and the walls are insulated with books. Books, books, and more books. I walked slowly through the nooks and crannies thinking about not just the stories between the pages, but the stories between the walls. What must have happened in this place? The people who must have passed through . . . It was like I was a kid again, lost in something beautiful. Greeted and enamored by the smell of aging books and fine champagne, my soul was happy. What seemed like a life never-ending, full of characters, prose, and food for thought, I felt the sudden urge to pee.

I brought Kelsey along to hold my glass of what I call "Titanic Champagne" and we chatted over the signed copy of *The Prince of Tides* tucked safely behind the glass in the fancy section. When it was my turn, I sprang into the bathroom and laid two strips of toilet paper down on the seat. In a flash, my mind went straight back to Granny's bathroom and the feeling of her mauve cushioned toilet seat under my heinie. The one I sat on my entire childhood, whether I was trying to escape a chore, hide from a pesty friend, or just really had to pee—the memories came flooding back.

I told Granny over and over that her pinchy seat cushion needed to go—that a few bucks would be money well spent for a new one, but she didn't seem to mind what she considered to be a minor inconvenience, as it was an otherwise perfectly good toilet seat. Now, with my heart and mind more open, memories like these are starting to come to me regularly. With Granny, I felt just like I did here in this bookstore, like the world is at my fingertips and I am free to do anything my heart feels like doing.

I can't help but wonder where memories like these were hiding all this time, and why I never felt the urge to tell someone. I can't help but think how sad it is that to avoid feeling pain, I've also avoided remembering. This, having these memories, the ones like the mauve toilet seat, is what makes me smile. This is what makes me excited about tomorrow.

This.

~Joy

For You (#TheLittleThings)

Dear Seeker,

Making sense out of your life isn't for the faint of heart, but if you've made it this far in the book, I'm sure you've already realized that. Understanding the Little Things is hard, and to be honest, I don't think I could have ever done it alone. Without the help of my therapist, friends to talk to, and opportunities to hear my own thoughts aloud, I'm not sure that I would have ever understood and accepted myself like I do now.

Without writing so much of it down on paper and giving myself the space to process it all, seeing the patterns and making connections, I might never have noticed the Little Things and the stories that I shared with you in this section. This kind of self-awareness is power. One that can be used for a better a life, healthier relationships, and more peace.

If I had known how to become more self-aware, maybe I would have heard the negative messages I carried around all these years, the ones that were too "little" to notice at the time—maybe everything could have been different.

Seeker, now is the time that I must ask you the questions. What messages, what Little Things, are you carrying around?

Think about these questions and create more of your own.

1. Do you remember a time when you said no to something you felt passionate about?
2. What was the last thing that you said no to, and what was the reason?
3. How often do you check in with your body before you make decisions? When is the last time you remember doing that?

Take a few moments to catalog those experiences.

4. What is something about yourself about which you are sensitive or ashamed?
5. What messages have you received about that thing?
6. What have you changed as a result?
7. How has that change caused you to feel?
8. As a kid, what were you praised for and what was shunned?
9. Were you told things were good or bad based on your gender?
10. Were you made to feel like your voice was not important? How early did that start?
11. Are there roads you avoid driving down? What do they make you think of?
12. What smells take you back to a moment in your past when you were flooded with emotion?
13. What associations do you make about things that others would never see?
14. What lengths do you go to so you can avoid these things?
15. How does that impact your relationships with others?

Those, Seeker, are the Little Things that are found in between the Big Things. Those are what we must open our eyes to—open our hearts to—because those little innocuous things are where we find meaning. They connect everything.

When I drew out my life, I could see from a bird's-eye view, and I finally began to understand this: **Big Things are easy to remember, but it's the Little Things that need to be recognized, because that is where joy is found.**

Kasey's Timeline

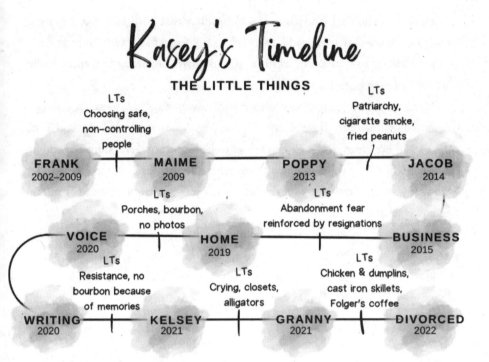

THE LITTLE THINGS

LTs
Choosing safe,
non-controlling
people

LTs
Patriarchy,
cigarette smoke,
fried peanuts

FRANK
2002–2009

MAIME
2009

POPPY
2013

JACOB
2014

LTs
Porches, bourbon,
no photos

LTs
Abandonment fear
reinforced by resignations

VOICE
2020

HOME
2019

BUSINESS
2015

LTs
Resistance, no
bourbon because
of memories

LTs
Crying, closets,
alligators

LTs
Chicken & dumplins,
cast iron skillets,
Folger's coffee

WRITING
2020

KELSEY
2021

GRANNY
2021

DIVORCED
2022

We all have hurt parts that need attention. But to find joy, you must throw away the idea that healing is forgetting—that the past is the past and looking back is foolish. Because it's not. It's the furthest thing from it.

Healing is understanding.

As long as you stay unaware of your feelings, you also stay unaware of things that trigger them. When Kelsey brought that suitcase downstairs, I immediately assumed that she was leaving. Of course, that wasn't true, but once I realized that a suitcase was a trigger for me, I was able to start the work to heal that wounded part of myself. That suitcase, that Little Thing, has such a bigger meaning, one that changes tons of tiny moments bound to make up the future.

The real result of healing is no longer reacting to old triggers (suitcases, closets, cigarette smoke) with the same intensity as before. The memories are still there, but they do not have the same power over your mind.

Healing is allowing yourself to feel things. It wasn't until I allowed emotions back into my life that I realized how much of my former self was controlled, not by me and what I wanted, but by my desire to prove something to someone who likely wasn't even paying attention.

Frank has never commented on my second marriage. He never mentioned my subsequent divorce. There was no "I told you so," no scathing lecture. All the things I had imagined him saying to me when he found out were completely in my head, but I had let it drive so much of my adult life that I'm ashamed to consider it now. It was like Frank took on the face of my fear of abandonment, but it, and it alone, is what drove things.

Live your life with one person's opinion in mind—yours. Pick back up your timeline and fill in the gaps with the Little Things as you begin to notice them. Just like you did before, notate each with your feelings. Was it traumatic, joyful, or something else? Don't be afraid to be vulnerable here. No one will see it but you.

Your Back Porch Bestie,

K

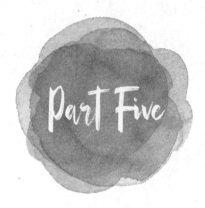

Change

THE OTHER SIDE OF FEAR

• Sometimes the place you are used
to is not where you belong. •

"We cannot become what we need to
be by remaining what we are."
~Max DePree

When I think of change, many things come to mind. Unfamiliarity and resistance are among them. Change is hard, but it is freeing. The following stories, all titled with a component of change, speak to the places change can hide in our lives and the light that change can bring if we're open to it. Immerse yourself in my evolution, and then search for your own. It is never too late to be what you think you could have been.

Courage

Change can only occur when awareness is present.

Why is it so hard?

Because we're scared.

So we run.

It's a conditioned trauma response, picked up from those who have modeled it for us. In short, it's familiar.

———

If you're anything like me, and I bet you are, you press on intently, setting your sights on the future, because if you're moving forward, you don't have to look back.

Looking back is exactly what I needed.

Not to revel in my misery or misfortunes but to understand myself better so that I could change *for the better*.

And I wholeheartedly believe that goes for you, too. It's okay to slow down. It's okay to idle. It's okay to look back.

Freedom from Fear

Colleagues in my professional circles call me a force. A machine.

"No moss grows on Kasey Compton," they say. "When do you sleep?"

I smile sheepishly, take the perceived compliment, and keep on truckin'. I don't believe them, though. I think I am just like everyone else. I think working from daylight to dark is something everyone does. But as I have become more aware of the meaning Little Things hold in my life, I realize my colleagues are right.

I am a force, but they don't know the whole story.

Through all my success, past and present, *fear* has been the *force* that drives me. My desire to avoid failure is so strong that the fear of it drives me to do more. My yearning to be loved, and my fear of someone realizing I am anything but lovable, pushes me to prove *it* wrong. Fear is what drives me to over-function, and as I come to understand and love myself, the question becomes, what will take *fear's* place? What does fear look like for you? Is it similar? Is it different?

If fear isn't my driving force, then what is?

———

"Can you see it now?" my therapist asks. "Can you see how all those Little Things led you here—the end of your relationship with Jacob, working on yourself through therapy, and reflecting on your past?"

I can. I've gone through the motions for so long, doing everything I thought I was "supposed" to do and denying my true self. I forced my feelings away, anything that would take me away from success; I buried them. What started in my mind, then moved through my heart, and manifested into my body as pain were Little Things.

My therapist helps me realize that my choice to leave my last relationship was valid. She helps me see that everything happening over the years that left me feeling hopeless is very similar to what I experienced growing up.

"I should have known our relationship wasn't going to last."

"Why is that?" she asks.

If I had been more self-aware, I could have understood my thoughts, feelings, and behaviors—the ones that I begrudgingly accepted—I would have known better than to believe that if someone loved me enough, *they* would change.

"I felt trapped. Financially, physically, mentally, and emotionally. And for me, when I'm trapped, I do one thing."

"Run," we both say in tandem.

Every time I acted out and made a wrong decision, it was because something or someone made me feel confined.

"There's evidence of that all over your timeline, isn't there?" she asks.

"Yep."

I feel a lack of control, fight, rebel, and then self-destruct.

"Self-sabotage?" she asks.

"Exactly. I've made a lot of terrible decisions. And when I'm alone without a support system, I think they're the worst mistakes ever—I beat myself up over them," I say. "So, as a result, more mistakes happen, all because I feel shame."

"And then what happens?" she asks.

"I make it worse. I *made* it worse," I correct myself.

Now, I realize that I once got hung up on shameful things and I let them control me, but everyone feels shame and regret.

"Have you learned anything over the last year in therapy?" she says.

"I've learned that I'm not alone in my fear. Many people are afraid of being unloved. A lot are afraid of failure. It's nothing to be ashamed of."

And fear doesn't have to be the force that drives me anymore. I can choose what that is. Whether it's joy, self-love, desire, or curiosity, the force that pushes me forward should always be up to me.

The therapist leans forward and smiles at me. There's a long silence, with the two of us looking ahead at the computer screen at one another. It's uncomfortable, but I embrace it. I breathe in slowly, then out, releasing all control to the universe.

Again, like I did nearly twelve months ago, I wonder if she sees any parts of herself in me.

Of course she does.

"This is called integration, Kasey," she says. "You're telling your story to me now with meaning, but you're not removed from it. Not like you once were."

She is right. I am not removed. I am not dissociating. I am not avoiding. I am owning. I'm changing.

"How does change feel?"

"*This* change feels good."

If you feel trapped by fear, one tiny step toward self-love can seem like a cross-country trek. It's easy to think there's too much work to do, that it's easier to stay where you are, to submit to your fears. But for change to occur, you must see fear for what it truly is. A liar.

We can only do better once we know. Fear and trauma are tricky in that they prevent us from understanding the events in our lives in a much deeper way. Acknowledging our past can be helpful, although it sometimes hurts. Sometimes it's that you need help seeing how the dots connect.

It's not to say that you can't, but it's certainly easier to go on this journey with support. Whether it's a family member, a bestie, or a therapist, it's easier not to go at it alone. If you've been thinking about change, and maybe, like me, you put it off for years, now might be the time to give therapy a try.

Reach out.

Make the call.

Defining Your Narrative

I've never admitted this to anyone.

I *am* sorry for hurting others, but I don't regret anything that happened. Not the two divorces, not the stint as a single mom, not being fired from a job, and not even filing for bankruptcy. It all sucked in the moment, and I thought my life was over with each situation, but it wasn't. It was only just beginning.

It was just the start of a new mindset. One filled with grit, perseverance, and determination—one that has become my backbone, keeping me strong, keeping me grounded. A mindset shaped by experiences, good and bad, which allowed me the opportunity for change. It is the start of wisdom, growth, and perspective. My fault or not, the things in my past gave me the ingredients for a fulfilling life, one overflowing with stability and love.

Without them, I could easily allow the traumas, big and small, to define me. I could end up like so many who tell themselves, "It happened for a reason." Living their life like they were only put here to experience this bad thing. Turning to addiction to numb the pain, tolerating unhealthy relationships to experience something that feels like home, and spending a lifetime trying to overcome the coping mechanisms that don't actually help you cope.

I don't believe bad things happen "just" for a reason. I don't think it is part of God's big plan. Trauma is awful. It will always be a part of you. But it doesn't have to define you. You don't have to tell others, or yourself, that it happened for a reason. You don't owe the bad things anything; you certainly don't owe them your joy.

Big Granny used to say, "It's just a messy kitchen, Kasey Renee." The food always tastes better when there's flour on the cutting board and dishes in the sink. You can appreciate the meal more when you know you worked hard to prepare it. The past is the past, and most of us hope it stays that way, but some live as if their past is their present—as if it controls them rather than just influences their choices.

For years after my parents' divorce, my mom lived like this invisible force was controlling her. Even though there was no going back, she carried the shame and guilt of it around until she married my stepdad when I was ten. He was certainly different from my dad, but there were characteristics he had as a husband that were more similar than I would have liked. I heard the stories Mom told me about her and Dad as they struggled through their relationship, and then I watched them play out again in many ways.

As a kid, I internalized her reaction to hardship and the shame of a failed marriage and financial struggles. When I went through a similar situation as an adult, I did precisely the same thing my mother did.

I repeated history.

I carried my past around like a backpack for a long time, keeping score of my mistakes and often sitting in judgment, too afraid to take it off, fearing that I might have to look inside. I kept my head down and tried to do my best, but I never felt like my best was good enough. I never felt like I was able to be free from my past.

I can't live that way *and* find joy—I must choose to change.

In many ways, especially as a child, I didn't have control over things that happened, and neither did my mom or you. But when we begin to understand ourselves, we can take back the control that we let shape us. We are the owner of how we connect the Little Things to the big ones. We have control over our awareness and how the pieces of the past fit together.

There's power in that. There's beauty in that.

You may not be able to change history, but you don't need to. You can use the people in your past and the events to learn and to grow. It's practicing acceptance without any excuses. This is when integration happens.

Yes, this happened to me. It was part of my past, but no, this does not define me, and it doesn't define my future.

Opening your eyes also opens your heart to your timeline and all the Little Things that fill in the gaps of the big events you call life.

And that, my Seeker friend, can change anyone.

Even you.

Let that shit go.

You deserve to be free.

Getting Honest

f we're being honest, as women, as humans, as people, we lie.

Yes, *we* lie.

I lie.

You lie.

All of us lie. But why?

It's not because we're bad. It's not because we're malicious. It's because we're afraid. We're afraid that if we tell the truth about the number of people we've slept with; whether we've had an abortion, been sexually assaulted, or been raped by a family member; or are having feelings for someone of the same sex, we'll be judged. We're afraid we'll be shamed, condemned, and abandoned. All of which reinforces humanity's biggest fears of failure and aloneness.

Shame is powerful. Shame is a silencer. Shame is a divider.

So we pretend we're good. We pretend we're happy. Tricking others and sometimes even ourselves, enough so to be a productive member of society—to blend in. But it's not sustainable and catches up to us in unsuspecting ways. Like at a book launch party.

Taking a good look at yourself, and not from a place of judgment but from a place of love, can mark the beginning of a transformation. What are you lying to yourself or others about, and why? What are you trying to protect yourself from? Is it your feelings? Are you lying about what makes you happy? Your past? It doesn't matter what it is, and you don't even have to tell anyone. It's just important that you know. *You* are the only one who matters.

This is not a conversation that you need to have with anyone but yourself or your therapist—I want you to know that. It's not even about *what* you are lying about, but about *why*.

It starts when we are groomed as children to feel shame. We're handed down this powerful behavioral modification tool by our parents, from their parents, going back who knows how long. We are programmed to protect our ego at all costs. It's a tactic to get a child to behave a certain way, whether intentional or not, and it causes us to choose: *us or them.* Unfortunately, more often than not, we choose them.

We choose everyone *but* ourselves.

Until we're tapped out. Until we're done. Until we can't go on one more day living a life that doesn't belong to us. Until we look around a house that we dreamed of owning, on a day we've always dreamed of experiencing, and realize that we feel nothing more than we did the day we filed for bankruptcy. We're just as empty as we were when we had nothing, even though, to outsiders, it looks like we have everything.

We is me.

We includes you.

My pretending disillusioned me.

And it will you, as well.

My lies caught up with me.

And they will you, as well.

And when they did, I chose honesty.

Not just to myself, but to everyone else.

And that, Seeker, was a gift.

One that smelled like roses.

And for the first time, they meant something different.

Because I was different.

What are you hiding? What lies do you tell yourself and the ones you love? What could someone else know that would cause you the most shame? Start there.

Maybe you're afraid of others, but what is that fear costing you? What are you compromising to save face for someone else?

Are you happy?

There's power in honesty.

Dare to live your truth, Seeker. I believe in you.

Be Vulnerable–August 2022

C an I tell you something?" I ask Kelsey as we lie sideways across what is now *our* bed.

She sits straight up and leans against the headboard. "Of course, baby."

I think back to a conversation we had some nine months back, her sitting across from me in my office, which made me realize something about happiness. She propped herself up against the right arm of the couch and sat quietly—more quietly than normal. My Granny was in the hospital from one of her falls, and Kelsey stopped by to see how I was doing.

Somehow, the conversation turned to what she dreams of, which made me think about my dreams. "Do you remember the time I asked you what you wanted out of life?" I ask.

I pause to look at her, gauge her recollection, and collect my thoughts. I can tell this conversation is catching her off guard, but it has been on my mind for a while.

The light that came in from the window behind her illuminating her face. Her eyes were a lighter shade of green that day, one that resembled my mom's. I saw a tear roll down her face.

"You were strong, but you were vulnerable and brave. So, I softened to you. I've never done that with anyone before."

At the time, I wondered what it was about my question that caused her so much pain. I was sorry. I felt this unrelenting need to protect her—to understand her.

"I encouraged you to tell me more. And you did."

"Yes, I remember," she says.

That day we talked about life, about living, about not settling—about going after your dreams and desires. It became clear that she had never even given herself permission to dream, probably like so many other women.

"That's when I knew why you seemed so sad. I didn't realize what was happening to me then. I didn't realize it until the day of the launch party that we were more alike than I ever imagined."

"I remember that tear," she says, "It had been years since I cried."

She sits up and repositions herself. I roll over with my head between my hands, so even when my eyes are open, all I see is the darkness of the comforter. I can't bear to look at anyone while sharing something so intimate. I trust her with my emotions, but I am still ashamed.

Back then my behavior was a way to cope. I thought joy only lived on the other side of success. But by then, I'd already developed maladaptive patterns, and getting shit done was a part of who I was. On the forefront, I was good—we were good, and my family was good, but underneath, I felt hollow.

"The best way I can describe this, which is probably not the greatest, is that I was digging away at myself so there was more space to work," I say. "And I didn't start to recognize it until I saw the pain in your eyes that day."

Years before all this started to unfold, I came home from work, got in bed, and slept alone nearly every night even though I was married to Jacob. While everyone else dreamed, I experienced twinges of sadness, then I'd start to dig. It was like I was scooping out all the feelings that slowed me down. The uncomfortable ones—the ones that made think—the ones that made me sad.

"My best friend, Karen, passed away while I was with Jacob, but I felt like I couldn't share my feelings with the person who was supposed to help carry my pain, so I removed them—I dug. One scoop at a time, one day at a time, I emptied my heart, soul, and all of myself, in front of the people who should have noticed a change in me."

I stop talking.

"But they didn't. They lived with me, worked with me, but never realized I was gone," I continue. "Kelsey. The scariest part of it all was that I had no idea what I was doing to myself. I didn't know I was digging so much and so often, emptying myself because I thought I had to. I could portray the loving wife, patient mother, and successful entrepreneur who had it all together when I had to. To do that, I'd lay the cover over my unearthed heart and carry on about my life, business as usual."

"You thought you had to *feel* nothing to *do* everything?"

"Pretty much. I didn't have the space for emotion."

I smiled and showed up for that event to raise money for the community. I put on my pearls and arrived early to that dinner. I laughed over a glass of wine and told a good story to the people at the table. I brought a bottle of Kentucky bourbon, thanked them for inviting me, and went home to pick up my shovel before I ever took off my party dress.

"I must have carried around painful memories but refused to process the feelings that went along with them."

Like when I needed affection and affirmation and didn't get it. Like when my parents were too busy fighting to realize that their daughter probably needed attention—even just one damn hug—but never got it.

So I dug. I allowed so much bullshit to happen, including that in my last relationship—I listened to all the excuses he made and settled for the crumbs and hated myself every day for it.

"One scoop at a time, one day at a time, I dug. And dug. And dug," I tell her.

Hearing the words come from my mouth lets loose another awakening. My body shudders, and I wrap my arms around myself as if to calm myself, while the tears seep from my eyes. They feel like weights, heavy with looming sorrow and regret. I must look broken and vulnerable—maybe a little brave, but sobbing, nonetheless. I feel the urge to run toward the closest closet, but I don't.

"I put on a happy front-facing exterior because I wanted the world to believe, me included, that everything was fine. If I had a way to cover it up, the emptiness I had hiding within me was my little secret, and I planned on keeping it that way forever."

She touches my arm, "It's okay. You can keep talking."

I feel safe now, so I do.

"When I listened to you talk about your life, I realized that mine wasn't so great either. I told you my marriage was fine because I wanted it to be, but it wasn't. After some soul-searching, I found the courage to lift up that cover and, for the first time, see what I had been doing all those years."

"I didn't think your marriage was fine," she says. "You say the people around you didn't notice *you* were missing, but I did. I didn't know you well enough to compare to how you once were, but there was more there. I could tell."

When your exterior portrays society's expectation of happiness, but your inside constantly feels alone and misunderstood, and everything around you affirms it, you start to question yourself. I always knew something was missing, something I'd been searching for, and finally it felt nice knowing that someone else noticed it, too.

"I wasn't sure I had the strength to do anything about it," I say.

I was tired. I was consumed with apprehension to face my deepest, darkest fear, but I knew I had to do it. I lost myself somewhere between the Big Things and the little ones and because of that, I was losing everything else in my life.

"It was like I took a deep breath, stood up on two feet, and pulled up the cover that was protecting all my vulnerabilities. I exhaled and forced my eyes down."

My chest hurts just telling her about it.

"What I saw was an image that I don't think I can ever unsee."

I pause.

"Kelsey, it was a grave. All those years, all those days, all those nights, I had been digging a fucking grave."

All my avoidance, the disregard of pain, and the distractions of life did this. I did this.

Every time I felt lonely, each time I felt disappointed, every moment I felt lost and found myself searching for the solution caused me to dig. I dug so much that by the time I realized my life wasn't working for me anymore, it was almost too late. The life I once knew was slipping through my fingers. This grave mirrored my future, especially if I didn't do something about it.

"I had no idea what was supposed to go there, but I had a feeling it was my hollow shell of a woman; after all, I didn't feel alive anyway. If I didn't do something, if something didn't change, I would be buried alive in a grave that I dug for my own damn self."

"You couldn't have done that much harm to your heart overnight," she says. "It would have taken years for that to happen."

The day I realized I lost myself was the day she and I had that first conversation in my office. I knew something had to change.

"I know I can never stop the fear, but I can stop letting fear control me," I say.

"It was a second chance, Kasey. Not everyone gets one of those," she says. "It was a wake-up call. Seeing that empty grave made you think. It made you change for the better."

I catch my breath and grab a drink of water.

The hard part is over.

To change, I must challenge everything that is comfortable. I must question what feels good in the moment for what is right for my joy.

"I never cried when Poppy died. Not when Granny died either. That's not normal, is it?" I ask.

She smiles. There's no need for words. I already know the answer. I think there is a part of me that knows if I start, I might not stop. There is something about looking down into that grave, though, that makes me think of Granny. It makes me think about Lennon. It makes me think about the meaning that *my* life carries. And my life can't have meaning without emotion.

The absence of vulnerability comes at a cost. For some, it's their family, their relationships, their connections. For me, it cost me all that, plus more. It took the empty grave to show me that. Was it worth it?

No. Now, the answer is clear. No.

Feelings are expensive, but they shouldn't cost you your life. And for me, the repressed memories, the walls built to defend the avoidance of conversations to keep from being hurt, nearly cost me everything.

"But it didn't," Kelsey says. "Your awareness saved you. Your desire to learn about yourself moved you from a place of uncertainty to one of confidence and change."

"It scared me to death," I say.

"Sometimes, that's what we need in order to feel alive."

―――――――

Maybe you've been hollowing yourself out for years. Maybe you've done it so long that that's all you know. The world likes to expect this of women, then blames them for not portraying the right amount of happiness.

We're either too much or not enough. Our expectations are too high, but if we don't settle, we're selfish. There's no winning.

The key here is to just stop. Stop digging away at yourself. Find what fills you up instead. Joy, self-love, freedom, creativity, passion, whatever it is. Give yourself more and more until you're overflowing. Never empty yourself again.

Grief—July 2022

On all accounts, the dust has settled. It's been nearly one year to the day since I filed, and my divorce is final. My children have adjusted well. I put my dream house up for sale and got an offer in the first week. I kept my businesses but sold the buildings they operated from. I have half as much money as I once did, and that's okay. At this very moment, I love myself a solid eight, teetering on a nine, and I am proud of that progress.

But there are times when I still grieve the old me, and I guess to some extent, I probably always will. Because of this journey to find joy, I realize that grief doesn't just happen when people die. Sometimes, we grieve the old version of ourselves—the person we once were, the one we've grown out of, the one that changed. Sometimes we grieve our old beliefs, even if they once led us astray. Sometimes, we grieve the illusion that we so heartily bought into, the one that told us that success *could* and *would* bring fulfillment.

Grief can happen when there's any kind of change, good or bad.

Saying goodbye to the old me, even though I like the new me so much more, is hard. *She* was a part of my life for a long time, and she still shows up sometimes in the Little Things. The triggers can light the fuse that causes me to revert backward, into old patterns, habits, and behaviors. That happened for years; the difference now is that I'm aware of it. I understand it. And I desire to change it.

So I pay attention.

Although I grieve, it's not because I miss *her* or want to be her again. I don't mourn the fence posts, but instead I can appreciate the fact that without *her*, I might not be *me*.

People expect me to be grateful that she is gone because I am better. But she *is* me, and I can't do that. I'll never regret who I once was, but that doesn't mean I don't feel pain sometimes. Right now, mostly, I feel hope.

And sometimes, I feel sorry.

Sorry I didn't see all of this before. Sorry that she had to endure so much heartache to understand that my Inner Child didn't have to live the way she lived. Sorry that she hurt and felt so lonely, and that I didn't know how to make it stop.

And that is grief—coming from a seedling, planted deep down in our hearts, and its name is Regret. We grieve what we "could have been," what we "should have been," and that we lost all that time in the process.

But, of course, all those years I thought I was searching for something and was running from fear, I just didn't know the path to find self-love and joy. I didn't know that all I needed was to find my way back home. To me.

Growing pains are still pain, even though it signifies healthy change. Grieving doesn't just stop, not even when you become the person you want to be.

Grief is an important part of this journey. Although most people don't look forward to pain, it's a necessary part of healing. Grief and pain are like sisters, connected by the very fibers that make them what they are.

Grief gives us the gift of perspective. Without perspective you can never achieve awareness, and without awareness, you can never understand your whole self. And there lies the pot of gold.

Perspective–April 2022

I live in a city with approximately five thousand people. The county, of course, is bigger, about seven hundred square miles with folks sprinkled out sparingly. Locals call it the Bible Belt of the South, where there's a church planted every hundred yards or so.

Most are avid Republicans; they construct large crosses on the highway to remind people that Jesus died on one and that they'll spend eternity burning in hell if they don't ask for forgiveness for their sins. Businesses are closed on Wednesday evenings and Sundays all day so parishioners can attend church. The typical family has a husband, a wife, 2.5 children, and a dog. We eat pinto beans with cornbread, onion, and a swirl of ketchup for family functions. We are known for our potluck dinners and southern hospitality.

I'm proud of where I'm from. I love the opportunity to raise my children here—a town that, for the most part, is safe. But I also know that I'm different from most of my neighbors on the outside. On the inside, I seriously doubt it.

I'm a nearly forty-year-old woman dating another woman almost ten years younger than me. I have a deep appreciation for bourbon and a newfound love for champagne. I believe in equality, and I love diversity. I always wanted a big, blended family in which the children didn't look like me. I believe in teaching them that love is love—that the color of their skin does not determine the kindness of their heart and that the person they bring home to meet me can be any religion, any gender, or any ethnicity.

Most importantly, I believe in acceptance, and I want my children and everyone else to know that. Because now, for the first time in my life, I have an inkling of what it feels like to be judged by strangers.

———

It's Easter Sunday, and Lennon is about to turn eight. She comes home from her dad's church and tells me she got saved. Ever since she was very young, she was curious about Christianity. As soon as she could talk, she'd quiz me on our morning drives to daycare about where we go when we die, if people are lonely buried in the ground, and whether our family members can see us from heaven. Sometimes she'd ask me things that I didn't know how to answer. I knew she was something special from the moment she was born, and conversations like these remind me of that.

We wait a year after she is saved before we talk about it again. I want to make sure she understands what she is committing to.

There's been a lot of talk about me around town. The split from Jacob and my relationship with Kelsey aren't anyone's business, but to some it's damn good tea to spill. I keep to myself throughout the whole thing, focusing on my own self-healing and love. The only people who know my side of the story are the ones who ask me directly. I can count those people on less than one hand. Yep, you read that right. No one asked me.

When Lennon announces her baptism date, I have mixed feelings. Grateful. Proud. But also terrified. Walking back into a church where I was once a member, where I once served, whose members have never reached out to me for the last year, is nearly debilitating.

I wear a blue dress with long sleeves and a high neck. It reminds me of something my grandma would like because it resembles a placemat. I take the whole family, Kelsey included, and we walk in proudly together. We are stared at together, we are judged together, and we are avoided together. Every moment

I stand awkwardly waiting to take our seats, I feel eyes on me—on us. I remind myself of why I am here: Lennon. She's really the only thing that matters.

I wince each time I walk past someone whom I used to call a friend but now who can't bear to acknowledge my existence. Each time they turn their head like they are looking for someone, I ache, because I know what they're doing. I notice the differences in my body, my breathing, and my energy.

I take a moment, out of the judgmental eyesight, and find the quietest place I can to center myself.

Don't give them the power.

You have no reason to feel shame.

You found yourself.

You love yourself.

You owe them nothing.

It helps, but it doesn't take away all the hurt, the flashbacks of rejection, and the years of religious trauma. It doesn't take me back to an unhealthy place like it very easily could. I don't avoid it. I don't dissociate from it. I feel it, and I breathe.

And when the lights go down and the music plays, all I can see is Lennon. My little blond-haired, blue-eyed, laundry-basket baby, becoming the person her heart is leading her to be. I have empowered her to do that, whatever *that* is. She knows that she can believe what she wants to believe and express it, and that I will always show up in support of her.

As uncomfortable as I am, I know I'm in the right place if I am close by, watching her. Even if it's in a place with people who once abandoned me, who were embarrassed of me when I tried so hard not to feel like an embarrassment to myself, here, being Lennon's mom, is the only kind of belonging I need.

I find joy here, even though I have prepared myself for a miserable morning and weeks of simmering drama after the fact. Even though I feel judged and unwelcome, joy is here, because my daughter is here, and she is happy.

I'll tell you the same thing I told myself. Write this down. Stick it in your pocket-book. Remember it.

> *Don't give them the power.*
> *You have no reason to feel shame.*
> *You found yourself.*
> *You love yourself.*
> *You have joy.*
> *You owe them nothing, Seeker.*

Communication–November 2022

"What's something you think you still need to work on?" my therapist asks about fourteen months into therapy.

I run through so many things in my mind. I have so much room for improvement, but at least I know that now.

What do I tell her?

"Communication," I say.

I've made so much more space for hard conversations over the last year, but it's still hard for me. It's hard not to revert to what's familiar.

"Do you have anyone who models healthy communication in your life?"

Should tell her about Kelsey? I know I'll have a lot of explaining to do, but this feels like the right time.

"Well . . . we're still working on it, but Kelsey and I are trying."

She's so patient with me. She, too, has wounded inner parts that cause her to fear confrontation in a different way than I do, but she pushes through. Sometimes I catch myself back in my old ways, allowing my triggers to take over, but we're improving. We are safe to one another, and that makes a difference.

"So, you two are *together, together* now?"

"Um . . ."

"You are, aren't you?" she asks.

I nod my head and smile.

"What's been the hardest part so far?"

"After all the work I've done on myself, I'd say the hardest part is recognizing and understanding each of our wounded parts and nurturing those through our relationship. Her tumultuous past relationships, my wounded Inner Child, we're trying to understand those in each other when we communicate."

"Wow, that's great. I'm proud of you," she says.

There it is again. Someone else told me they are proud of me.

I'm proud, too. When they say relationships take work, I see that now. What we are doing is certainly work, but there's also a lot of love there. She's my best friend.

"Hey, Kels, I met with my therapist today," I say as she barges through my office door. This time, there's no hesitation when she visits me. She walks straight up to where I sit and kisses me softly on the mouth.

"Oh yeah, what'd she know?"

"More than me," I giggle.

"You tell her about us yet?" she asks.

"Well . . ."

Kelsey and I talk about our therapy sessions each time we have one. We jokingly call it de-briefing, but it really is how we process therapy so we can understand each other a little more.

"In the spirit of communication and curiosity, can I ask you something?" I ask. I don't wait on a response because I'm afraid I'll lose my nerve.

"Remember back before my book launch when you asked me for a therapist recommendation?"

She looks nervous.

"You said you had some things you needed to sort out and thought you needed some help," I say. "What *did* you need help with?"

She shifts her position at the other end of the couch and sits up with both feet touching the floor. She moves her hands to her knees and rocks slightly while the quietness swallows us. The longer I sit, the more nervous I get. I brace myself for something I might not want to hear. I don't know if I can handle sharing more of her pain, her trauma, anything that would cause me to hurt for her.

"*You, Kasey.* I couldn't stop thinking about *you.*"

"Wait. You wanted to go to therapy because of me. You barely knew me."

"Yes, I couldn't get you out of my head, but I was never going to tell anyone—especially not you."

"What changed your mind?" I ask.

I think I know, but I wait for her to continue.

"You were bold that day, do you remember that?" she asks.

"Not really. It's a little bit of a blur."

"You looked me straight in the face and said, 'What are your intentions with me?'"

Oh. I did say that.

I couldn't keep quiet about the tension. There was something there, and I'd never experienced anything like that. Especially not with a woman. If I were being honest with myself, I liked Kelsey, but I never thought those feelings would be reciprocated.

"I asked why you were asking," she says.

"Yeah, you kept answering my questions with questions."

"I was nervous," she says. "You mentioned meeting in the office in the hallway, the time in Gatlinburg, the birthday celebrations we were both a part of, the green high heels," she continues.

Now my mind is racing. I did mention all these things; they were all Little Things that were etched in my memory and caused me to think that meeting Kelsey was not an accident.

"I thought about every single one of those things, too. For years. Nights, I'd sit up in my recliner watching TV, thinking about them. About you."

I did the same thing. The what-ifs. What it would be like to be close to her, to touch her arm, to breathe her in.

"And when you listed them out, it was like *you* were the mirror. I knew it was *you.* I knew you were the one I was meant to live my life with," she says. "I cried that day because you made me feel safe. I cried, Kasey, because I knew there was no going back. My life was going to change forever."

I knew that, too. There was no way it couldn't. She opened my eyes to see a life that I was letting pass me by in a lot of ways. Whether I ended up with her or not didn't really matter because I could see. And when you *know better*, you must *do better*, right?

I knew I had to get a divorce.

I knew I had to feel joy.

I knew my kids needed a more present mother.

I knew that life was going by too fast.

I knew that I had so much more to live.

I knew that I wanted to feel something.

With someone.

Maybe with *her*.

———

You should feel joy.

Your kids need a more present parent.

Life goes by fast.

You have so much more to live.

You deserve to feel something.

So go, feel, *live*.

Self-Trust–June 2022

Trusting yourself means loving yourself.

Loving yourself is letting go of the feelings attached to the opinions of others. Self-love is freeing.

A few months into this process, I get a text from a friend I haven't spoken to in nearly twenty years.

"Hey. I saw your Facebook post. It's been a while, so I don't know what's going on in your life, but you said something about a journey of self-exploration and self-love. I've been where you are. I feel compelled to warn you. Everything is about to change. The people who were once in your life may no longer be there after you do this. But in the end, the only one that matters will be—*you*. You'll find yourself, and that will be worth all the weight of the loss."—Nate

The text paralyzes me. I don't respond for a couple of days because, to be honest, I don't know what to say. He is probably right, but I am not ready to deal with more loss. I need to trust myself first, my decisions, my feelings, and my heart.

———

Trust in another person is the foundation for any relationship, even the one we have with ourselves. We often forget that. We are not taught to trust, which takes time, trial, and experience. Trust takes listening to our body, being attuned to our feelings, and acting on our instincts. Trust and love go hand in hand.

Trust requires love. It's messy, but it sets you free.

Trust is related to triggers.

A trigger is activated by a wound.

Wounds are hurts, etched in our memories.

Memories activate the triggers.

We react to triggers, either in a healthy way *or* an unhealthy one.

Your ability to trust becomes contingent on your timeline and what is found there.

In the Big Things, in the pain, and in the hurt.

Look at the big events and markers in your life and ask yourself if there are any that caused *you* to mistrust. An instance when someone hurt you or let you down? What reminds you of that hurt? *That is a trigger.* What is your body's response to that memory, to that trigger? What do you do? *Those are the Little Things.*

Remember, your happiness is not contingent on someone else; it's contingent on you, and your ability to love and trust yourself.

Self-Love

When we get down to the root of self-love, we should first look at what it is not. It is not self-sabotage in any form—it is the opposite. There's only one reason a person continually makes choices that harm themselves, over and over and over again. And that is because they don't love themselves. For a long time, I didn't love myself.

At times, I hated myself and didn't know how to move past it. I imagined I'd live the rest of my life that way, so I pretended I was fine the way I was.

To be "fine" means that something will always feel like it's missing. You'll carry on business as usual, but there will be a void. A hole. Maybe a grave. My "fine" led me to search, and I filled that void with romantic relationships, children, pets, a career, a dream home, a vacation home, and everything I could chase.

The problem was that the void was still there.

I thought it was a lot of things, but all along, that thing that was missing was joy. I didn't know that. I also didn't realize that the only way to find it is to first love myself.

Loving myself meant letting go of the old beliefs, the unhealthy inner voice that told me I was not enough, that if I was not perfect, I would be alone. It meant swallowing my pride, to be honest with myself about how I truly felt. To release the shame and own my mistakes.

Loving myself meant setting boundaries for people in my life, like Victor, who served as a symbol of my own self-sabotage. It meant finally coming to terms with Frank, who was the face of my fear, and forgiving myself for hurting him. It meant receiving flowers from Kelsey for no reason other than she saw them, and they reminded her of me.

Loving myself means holding space for others' feelings, even if I don't understand or agree with them. It means hearing words I don't necessarily want to hear and compartmentalizing them in a way that doesn't break me down. It means sitting with my children when they cry, curious about their hurt, but letting go of the need to fix it.

Loving myself means still having questions about why Jacob didn't tell me things, why he lied, and why he stayed, but respecting myself enough not to ask. Loving myself enough to let it go, to move forward because hearing the answer won't change anything.

I've come to realize that self-love and joy are connected much like Granny and Poppy; you can't have one without the other. You can't have a tough conversation without a ham salad sandwich. You can't take a Sunday evening drive without beef jerky and orange soda. Some things are just better together.

———

Seeker, how much do you love yourself? At what point, at what number (remembering how I went from a two to an eight), does loving yourself feel different? What does your self-love, or lack thereof, look like? What feels like it's missing? Is it joy? Is that something you could use more of?

If so, how much do you love yourself on a scale from one to ten? Don't be ashamed of your answer. My "two" all those months ago was brutal, but it was brutally honest as well. I needed to acknowledge how far I had to go before I could commit to starting my journey.

If it's anything less than a ten, you have some work to do, my friend.

Changing—August 2022

Dear Journal,

My therapist told me to book a trip to Portugal for twelve months after our first session. Here we are over a year later, and I still haven't booked it, but I'm close.

I'm to a point now where it's not so much about looking back but forward. It's what I want from my one shot at life, and I don't mean happiness, because of course I want that. Everyone does. I mean what I want in a relationship, how I want to be treated, how I want to show up for my kids, and the feelings I want to experience on a regular basis.

I'm different now. Instead of more, I want less for the first time: a smaller office, less bills, fewer responsibilities, less distractions. I want to serve my clients and readers, but not in excess, not at the expense of joy—not if it means sacrificing energy that I have already reserved for myself and the ones I love.

I want to wake up and see if my succulents have sprouted any babies because that makes me smile. I want to bake peach cobblers and let my kids help me measure the sugar and flour. I want to put my baby boy in cute pajamas each night and read him a book before bed. I want to walk and talk to Lennon about honesty and her feelings. I want to crawl into bed so I can lie on the chest of the first person I've felt safe enough to let see me, the person who makes me feel wholly loved.

I want to travel and enjoy every part of the journey. I want to experience new things with people, be immersed in the moment, and not be afraid of the feelings that follow. I want to talk about real things with someone who hears me. I want to use the skills I've learned over the last year to understand others and use conflict to deepen relationships rather than letting it destroy. I want to break the dysfunctional cycle that I was raised in.

This newfound awareness allowed me to make space for emotions. That's what I was lacking. But not anymore. When I see myself now, I see more than this hollow shell hiding from the world, fearing just as much to be seen as to be forgotten. In me I see Poppy and his meticulous ways, the ones that gave me the character traits for the success I've had in business. The lessons I took from him, like drawing it out, led me here.

Granny and her memories gave me something to look back on and look forward to. As for Mom, the woman I got my strength from, my work ethic, and my ferocious protection for my children, she helped me break a cycle that desperately needed breaking. My Old Man is still a bit of a mystery, and there's a lot that I can't make sense of right now, but he taught me the importance of quality time and what that means to a child.

The combination of all these people gave me enough understanding to make an impact. I just needed the space to see and receive it.

~Changing

For You (#Change)

Dear Seeker,

For years I thought I was fine—I dealt with all my heartaches and hard times and was "over it." But clearly, I wasn't. And I don't think most of us are. Let's be honest with ourselves: we weren't taught to process emotions as children, and we certainly don't learn as adults.

Emotions are hard, they're scary, they're confusing, but they're necessary. For love, for forgiveness, for understanding, for grace, for perseverance, for grit, for everything, we need them. I recently interviewed Jessica Schroeder, an Emotionally Focused Therapist (EFT) out of Kansas City, Kansas. She described avoidance as a common relationship that people have with pain, and I've been a front-row participant in that.

If you find yourself avoiding pain, you may still be stuck in a Big Thing, where an unhealed part keeps showing up in Little Things. To move past that pain and level of "stuckness" and into a place of integration, to a place where you can change, you must focus on your ability and willingness to see.

Pull out your notebook and look at both the Big and Little Things. Then ask yourself, what keeps showing up? Where do I continue to get stuck? Mark those areas with a big black X and write out as much as you feel comfortable about the stuckness you're experiencing. Then ask yourself what it is you might need to move forward. For me, it was emotional safety.

Maybe it goes back to the good ole limbic system, the one that wired our bodies for safety. Perhaps my body got confused somewhere in my timeline; I confused familiarity with safety, but now I have learned that just because something feels familiar or comfortable, it's not always safe.

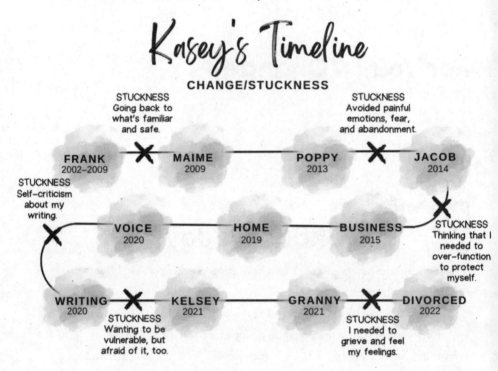

Kasey's Timeline

CHANGE/STUCKNESS

STUCKNESS
Going back to
what's familiar
and safe.

STUCKNESS
Avoided painful
emotions, fear,
and abandonment.

FRANK 2002–2009   **MAIME** 2009   **POPPY** 2013   **JACOB** 2014

STUCKNESS
Self-criticism
about my
writing.

VOICE 2020   **HOME** 2019   **BUSINESS** 2015

STUCKNESS
Thinking that I
needed to
over-function
to protect
myself.

WRITING 2020   **KELSEY** 2021   **GRANNY** 2021   **DIVORCED** 2022

STUCKNESS
Wanting to be
vulnerable, but
afraid of it, too.

STUCKNESS
I needed to
grieve and feel
my feelings.

Physical safety is easy to understand, but emotional safety is a key component needed to achieve awareness and understanding, one I never even knew about until Kelsey came along. Your body, mind, and spirit know if you are not in a safe environment, one that would not accept or support your thoughts and feelings. You can't fully step into understanding if you're guarded, because that is the opposite of vulnerability, and vulnerability calls for you to be brave.

Sometimes this means setting boundaries or changing the level of access you give people. It might mean you have to tighten your inner circle, say no when you're used to saying yes, and take more time for yourself than you usually do.

What you do with it now—how much you change, how much you "un-stuck yourself," how much you grow, how much you run toward joy—that's all up to you.

Your Back Porch Bestie,

K

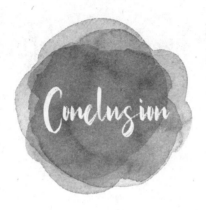

Choosing Joy

• It's not through healing that you will love yourself. It's through loving yourself that you will heal and be joyful. •

"When joy is a habit, love is a reflex."
~Bob Goff, *Everybody, Always: Becoming Love in a World Full of Setbacks and Difficult People*

Joy comes from a safe, secure, and healed Inner Child. It never leaves you; it just needs to be tapped into again.
So, tap, tap, tap, Seeker.
Remember *her*.
Understand *her*.
Then allow *her* the space to change.
Give *her* the room for joy.

What I Am—March 2023

It's been a while since I last saw you," my therapist says.

It *has* been a while—eighteen months since our first session. So much has happened in that time. I bought a new house. I bought land to build a forever home on and restarted my life with a softer side. I tied up loose ends, put some fears to bed, and felt less resistance in turning back toward my past, and certainly less about what's to come in my future.

"I know," I say. "Life got busy!"

"Well, fill me in."

"It's all starting to come together," I tell her.

I'm happy—actually, happy. I'm less productive now than I've ever been, but I'm okay with it. I make less money now than I have in years, but I'm okay with that, too. I'm okay with all the changes in my life.

"I feel lighter."

Sure, there are still some regrets. There are still a few what-abouts and what-ifs. There's still some baggage I carry, specifically about failure, and about letting people down, but there's also love and grace and peace, and that's never been there until now.

"Lighter, how?"

"Less serious. More playful. More in the moment." I pause, letting my own words sink in. "More like a child."

A smile beams across her face.

"You've found joy."

I *have* found joy in everything. From cooking breakfast on Sunday morning, to propagating plants. I have found joy in decorating my current home, and in building my forever one. I have found joy in watching my baby boy play T-ball. I have found joy in asking Lennon what she's feeling. I have found joy in watching Maime come into her own and meeting her needs in the way that I wish mine had been met. There is joy in my life now, and it's all around me.

"You've found self-love, too," she says.

I still love myself a solid eight these days. Some days feel like a ten, and others like a six, but never a two like it once was.

"Yes, it feels like I've found me again."

"And who did you discover that you are?"

I think long, deep, and slowly, but the words enter my mind as if they'd been there all along.

"I am many things. But above all, I am fulfilled."

"And that is enough," she says.

"And that is enough," I repeat.

Our session comes to a close, and she asks, "Can you give me a status update on a few things really fast?"

"Sure," I say.

"Frank?" she says as if it is a question.

"Forgiven."

"Victor? she says.

"Victor, who?" I chuckle.

"Jacob?"

"Free. Almost entirely free."

"And Kelsey?"

"Loved. Unconditionally loved."

She smiles. I smile. No other words are said.

I AM SAFE AND FREE

Loving yourself changes things.

Ten years ago, I craved the ocean with every fiber of my being. I'd sit on the sand and look out toward the horizon, because it made me feel free, and that's what I wanted. Freedom. I thought money, success, and a beach house would give me the feeling I was looking for, but it didn't.

And I didn't know why.

I still love the ocean, but I don't crave it like I used to. Maybe because I no longer need *it*, something out there, to fill a void. I was never trapped because of a failing marriage, because I once lived in poverty, or because I lacked the support that I needed to be better. I was trapped somewhere much more dangerous, inside my own soul, running from fear, and searching for something that I could never find "out there."

Now I'm happy being home. Sometimes I think about curling up in front of a fire, in a tiny cabin surrounded by mountains. I've spent a lot of time wondering why. I think it's because in my heart that means safety. Since I no longer feel the need to be free, all I want is to be safe and to be loved.

When I am safe, I *am* free. When I am safe, I can be vulnerable. When I am safe, I can be anything, I can be all things, I can be everything I want.

———

When I called Tara in late 2021, freshly separated, confused, frazzled, and unsure about my feelings for Kelsey, she summed it up for me in two words, words that I had never heard used together—words that were as foreign to me as the people of Portugal.

Emotional safety.

It caused my gut to wake up and my insides to listen. They made me question my friendships, previous relationships, and the history of interactions I had with family members. They sparked even more questions about who I am as a woman, how I view men, and how I fit into a community of people I perceive as strangers.

She spoke as if it were easy, as if the answer to my questions was one that she had answered hundreds of times or more. She was confident in her approach but empathetic to my lack of ability to see.

"Have you ever really trusted anyone?" she asked me.

"Yeah, I think so."

"Do you remember who the last person was?"

"I was nineteen. It's been twenty years."

"You don't have to tell me, but think about that time. That person. Think about what happened and what you lost. How you hurt. How you changed. Think about that, and you will learn a lot about why you feel the way you feel now," she said.

This was not on my timeline; it was too painful to put on there, even though so much time has passed.

But I knew what she meant. The first person I ever truly trusted with my heart did something to it in such a disgusting and isolating way. Something that caused me to build walls, force out vulnerability, and harden my exterior for so long that my heart also began to harden as well. That never changed, not with Frank or Jacob, or anyone until I felt safe with Kelsey. Then I felt free to be me.

———

When we are safe, joy can be tapped into—like a reservoir. It's like a body of water, something we can't live without, something that feeds our being, something that proves that we're alive—we just need to know where to find it. We must know where it lives. We must have the space in our hearts to see. We must have the tools to access it. Like all things, it wants to be needed.

We all have this reservoir; some go a lifetime without it; some find it when they're young and hold on to it forever; some play a game of hide-and-seek, experiencing twinges of joy off and on over the years. It's never too late, because it never goes away; it sits there patiently waiting and watching to see what we are going to do with it. It never turns its back on us.

I spent my life searching for something to fulfill me—looking for that feeling because I needed it to feel alive. I just didn't know where it was or how to use it, even when it was within me all along.

Joy, Seeker, embraces peace and contentment. Joy is present when others may see no reason for it to be there; it needs no escape, no search, because it can be felt anywhere, with anyone, at any time. Not just at Granny and Poppy's house, on vacation, or in a hotel room holed up to write a book. Joy, unlike happiness, does not need to be chased, pursued, or searched for.

Joy transcends; it's carried within our soul from one person we love to the next. It's felt by our children, lovers, and those around us whom we choose to let see. It seeps from our pores, glowing across our faces. Joy, in some regards, is expensive, especially if we spend our lives searching for it. We buy new cars, build houses, and revel in all the toys life offers, only to come up short. We end marriages, change our identities, and sometimes start entirely over just to take a different path that will bring us closer to the feeling we are after.

Joy is priceless, though. And once you feel it, you will want more. It will help you shape your thoughts; it will help you choose yourself over them. Joy will stack the deck in your favor; it will cause you to want more, but always in a good way. It is wholesome and pure and won't steer you in the wrong direction. It can unleash an awakening within your body that changes the way you look at others. The tension that once burdened your muscles will not be as strong, and within you, you will create more space to love.

Loving yourself leads to joy, and joy makes room for more love. It increases your tolerance window and allows you to reset from stress and the anxieties that fill your head. It allows you to find peace and comfort in a person who, by all accounts, never seemed like someone you would or could ever fall in love with.

We are all different, and we all experience it in ways that are unique to us, but for me, joy gave me my life back. It gave my kids their mom back. The pain I experienced gave me a new perspective on life, strengthened my purpose, and made all the good things even better. It caused me to slow down and experience moments rather than just waiting for the next thing to happen—the next weekend to come, the next vacation to go on, or the next surge at work to require all my attention. Joy is an addiction that I don't have to feel bad about—one I will never have to recover from, one that surpasses a Band-Aid for my hurts. Now when I feel the need to search for something, it doesn't have to be a shiny object, or success, or a distraction. Now all I search for is awareness, understanding, and joy.

But mainly, just joy.

I AM JOY

Sitting there in my bourbon cabinet is a ceramic alligator painted a playful teal. I put it there for safekeeping, but it doesn't belong to me.

It's hers. It's Kelsey's.

We live together now. We started fresh with a house that has no negative ties to the past, and we decorated it with things that are meaningful to us. Every time I see that little gator, I hear Kelsey's voice in my ear, just like we are still there in Beaufort, that late fall afternoon.

"What if we paint something for each other?" Kelsey asks.

Overwhelmed by options as we enter the front door of a paint-your-own-pottery shop, I spin around to take it all in. Old wooden shelves, probably a hundred years old, hold all the figurines, pots, mugs, and planters, on three out of the four walls. Divided into groups by holidays, new babies, sports, and the like, there are so many to choose from. Everything is white, unpainted, and pure—ready to absorb all our creative energy with a brush stroke.

"Sure."

At first glance, nothing catches my eye. Honestly, I am overwhelmed by the sheer volume of whiteness. And painting something for Kelsey is different from choosing something for myself. I want it to have meaning because she will appreciate that. I need to take my time and find something perfect.

"Hey, girls, ya'll sisters?" the shop owner asks when she spots us from where she is standing near the kiln.

We smile politely and look at one another. Kelsey waits for me to answer, like she always does.

"Something like that," I say.

I don't need to define the terms of our relationship to the old lady who runs the paint shop, so I don't. Maybe it is just that, or maybe it is something more. Maybe I haven't quite come to terms with how *I* define it, which makes it hard for me to explain it to someone else.

I can't sum it up in a word, or five, or even ten. I don't know if it bothers her, but I regret it, immediately.

"Well, come on over and let me explain how this here stuff works."

She is sweet and reminds me of Big Granny. Welcoming, friendly, and curious—she wants to know everything about us. Where we are from, what we are doing down in the Lowcountry, and why we decided to stop in for a paint.

I use this as a step toward redemption. I tell her about our kids, how *we* have four, including Kelsey's—three are mine, one is Kelsey's, but they are all *ours* now. I include the word *we* as often as I can, like how "we" are a family, and "we" are together.

It doesn't take Kelsey long to grab a flower vase from the shelf, and she is off, picking out colors and sitting down to start her design. I know why she wants to paint that for me. She knows I love flowers; she knows the meaning they used to have in my life, and she knows what they mean now. She wants to celebrate that change.

But me? I still don't know what to choose.

"Girls, I hate to do this, but my little grands will be here in right about forty-five minutes, so I'll need you to wrap up by then, if that's okay?"

We can't argue with that. *Grandkids come first.*

I move around the shop feeling the pressure from the clock up above the window, looking up and down, waiting for something to speak to me. A little white dog catches my eye first. Kelsey doesn't like dogs, but this one gives me pause, and I don't know why. Steadily, I move closer, noticing details that I didn't see at first.

A familiar feeling washes over my body. It starts with my feet and moves up like a riptide pulling me under water. My heart races, my face feels flushed, my head seems to swim around the room. The tingling in my fingertips is the only thing that allows me to resist the urge to pick it up; after all, I don't want to break it.

I want to know more about it, though: what it is bringing up for me, and why I feel the way I do in this moment. And within the milliseconds that must have passed, it is like I am transported back to the living room in my old house the night of my book launch. At a time in my life when I should have felt joy and didn't, I remember scanning the room for anything that would ground me before my guests saw me at my worst. It brings me back to the moment when my eyes land on those cement German shepherd bookends, when I felt guilty for not feeling grateful.

But standing there in that paint shop, I experience a similar feeling, almost as if I am outside of my own body again. Unsure about what is real and what isn't. It is like two lives—one old, one new—running parallel, never touching, just waiting for me to choose.

This or that?

Present or past?

I know, without a shadow of a doubt, what to choose. Not what's easy, not what's familiar, but what challenges me—what makes me better, what serves me on the inside. It left me once again thinking about Frank, and how I outwardly chose everything to chase after—but not this time.

The choice leaves me thinking about the work it took to get to where I am, to a place where joy could be tapped into easily, where seeing a ceramic dog could fill my heart with love and thankfulness.

Nothing "out there," nor nothing on those custom built-ins of my past dream home, sparked a desired feeling, a memory, or a story—they brought about nothing that I thought they should. But there, in the little paint shop off Ribaut Road, I smile looking at a dog. I smile looking at a monster truck my son would like if he were here. I am having fun. I am doing something trivial, but I am happy.

Kelsey starts painting nearly twenty minutes before me because I am lost in the memories, lost in the feelings, trying to find something perfect—simple and understated. I think about our relationship and imagine what a perfect symbol of our love might be if there is such a thing.

I can't tell you why, but when I see *something* lurking in the corner, as alligators tend to do, I know. Not much bigger than the palm of my hand—it must be *her*. We'll call her Alice. Small and dainty, but ferocious all at the same time. Protective, quiet, and delicate. Thoughtful, intentional, and beautiful. She doesn't need painting, but I pick out a color anyway since that's what I am there to do.

As the brush strokes take over me, and music plays in the background, Kelsey's green eyes peer at me from across the table. I travel off again to a place in my heart, thinking about how two years ago I would not be doing this. After some time, I'm not sure how long, I look down at my teal alligator and realize I am doing nothing more than painting a piece of ceramic, but I am fulfilled.

The faint sound of music in the background perfectly collides with my feelings. It's not too loud; it's not too soft—it is just right. Kelsey means the world to me. I also know, at this point in my life, I would still feel content if I was sitting here painting alone. This is what I have been working toward—self-love—and that's what I have finally achieved. It is better here with her, though.

Each time I open the door to my bourbon cabinet, I still think about alligators and why Alice spoke to me that day. Maybe it's because alligators are one of the oldest surviving species on the planet, and that's what I want from my relationship.

Maybe it's because they're known for their instincts, and mine took me straight to Kelsey. Once my eyes connected with hers for the first time there in the hallway of my office, I could never pry them away. Kelsey's all I see; she is love, she is peace, *she* is home. *My* home, no matter where we are.

Like an alligator, on land or in water, with her or by myself, at home or somewhere else, I know where joy lives.

Joy lives in me. And joy can live in you.

I AM LOVED

All my life I've had trouble saying those three words: "I love you."

I feel them, deeply. But getting them out is another thing entirely. I struggled to say them to Maime when she was born, but once I did, I knew I meant it.

I'm thirty-nine now. I can't remember the last time either of my parents told me they loved me, so I stopped expecting it. I told myself I didn't need it, but those wounds stuck around. Each time we hung up from a phone call or left a family event, I waited to hear it, but there was silence instead. Over time, calluses formed on my heart. The hurt lessened each time because my heart was numb.

On February 1, 2023, the day I turned thirty-nine, I received a text that I will keep forever.

"Happy Birthday. I love you. I am proud of you."

My family hasn't celebrated my birthday since I was a little girl. No birthday cakes or presents, but sometimes the Old Man gets me a card.

"Kelsey, you're not going to believe what just happened," I say.

"What?" she says with excitement.

I take the phone, open it to the message thread, and stick it in front of her face.

"Your mom?" she asks.

"She told me she loves me."

"Are you going to respond?"

That is a good question. *Am I?*

———

Of course I am.

I'm not the same person I was two years ago. I am better at accepting help and being vulnerable. I couldn't give the kind of love I want for myself unless I'm able to understand it and accept it. It feels different to have emotional tolerance for love and affection—Kelsey helped me with that; therapy helped me with that.

Now I'm ready. I understand love so much better. I understand my mom so much better—the way she poured all of herself into everyone else, never giving herself a chance to heal. I know she needs to hear the same things I've had to tell myself over and over the last two years.

You are going to be okay.

You are not alone.

You are safe.

Seen.

Heard.

Loved.

"Hey Mom, I love you, too. Thank you."

I lay my phone on my chest, close my eyes, and fall asleep.

Ten—July 2023

Dear Journal,

There are so many things I could say here, two years post-book launch, but I think I can narrow it down to just a handful:

    Passport application complete.
    Passport application submitted.
    Portugal flights booked.
    Ten.
    I love myself a ten.

~Me

For You (#ChooseJoy)

Dear Seeker,

If you would have asked me ten years ago to write a story about what my life would look like now, it certainly wouldn't have been this one. Would I have told you that my two serious relationships would end in divorce? *No.* Would I have three kids and be considering more? *Probably not.* Would I feel deeply connected in an intimate way with a woman? *Hell no.*

But here I am, throwing the last bit of convention right out the window, living my life in a way that feels right to me. Not caring about what others think, noticing my Inner Child showing up in interactions from my day, and loving it. Here I am, committed to feeling emotions and accepting them, and all the other things I cannot change. I'm here doing things that I was once too afraid to even consider.

I love myself despite my mistakes, despite my failures, because I know my intentions are good and my heart is in the right place. I'm well aware that people will draw their own conclusions, and many of those may not include accepting me, supporting me, or believing in me, and that is okay.

I am here because even though looking back and remembering takes effort, it is worth it. Increasing awareness of my own thoughts, feelings, and behaviors took hard work and perseverance, but I was dedicated to it. Opening up in therapy to work toward the change I wanted to see in my life was exhausting, but I did it, and so can you.

I am here now, a different person, because change occurred. I am here, filled with joy, because change occurred. Because I sought understanding. Because I gained awareness. I am here, filled with joy, because I started to remember—because for once, I searched for me.

You are here, too, friend. Journal in hand, think about how far you have come and how far you can still go. At this point in your search, I want you to think about moments in your life *now* that resemble those from your childhood. Moments when you feel free, silly, or curious.

Write them down. Here are some examples that I wrote for myself.

- Having a water balloon fight with the kids on Saturday.
- Taking a detour for ice cream when it's late and already past my bedtime.
- Catching fireflies on the first warm night of summer.

Now answer these questions:

1. Did you have a lot of moments on your list, or do you wish there were more?
2. If you had to label one thing as the reason you don't have more of these childlike moments, what would it be?
3. What could you do to rid that barrier to these joyful moments?

Joy is ultimately a choice, but it might not have been when you first started this process. It becomes that way once you have the space in your mind, in your heart, and down deep in your bones, to accept it—to choose it, to embrace it. Joy is wherever your Inner Child is, which is why I wanted you to start by finding *her*. When you know where she is, when you can tap into her emotions, you become closer to your truest self.

I don't know what the future will hold for me. I don't know if I'll ever get married again, and if I do, there's no way to know how it will end. I don't know if I will be with the same person until the day that I die. I don't know any of those things, and for the first time ever that feels okay. I accept the unknown, along with my growth, my new perspective, and the sense of home I now feel within myself. It's a calming feeling, one that gives me hope. One that I know will prevent me from baking whole cookies or accepting the crumbs. My self-love grounds me, and that inner whisper says something different than it used to.

It says, *you deserve better.* It says, *you're going to be okay.* It says, *you are loved.*

Self-love trumps fear, always.

The changes for you will be undeniable. Despite all the challenges of change, you will grow. You will persevere. If you hang in there, even when all you want to do is let go, you will find what you're searching for.

Whatever is in the way of joy, whether it be childhood trauma, adulthood trauma, fear, avoidance, triggers, anger, or self-sabotage, know they're just barriers. They may feel big in the moment or when your Inner Child is still wounded, but they're just bumps, roadblocks, and detours on the path toward an untapped reservoir of joy waiting for you.

Now, there's no need to walk in with rose-colored glasses, desperately hoping that someone will love you and fix whatever is broken inside of you. Now, you no longer must think that if only you are good enough, someone will stay.

Now, because you have yourself to always fall back on, you can trust that what happens is meant to be.

Your Back Porch Bestie,

K

P.S. As this book and these conversations have progressed, Kelsey and I thought there was much more to be said about self-love, joy, and fulfillment. Find yourself wanting to explore more internally? We'd love for you to check out our podcast, *The Back Porch Bestie,* and interact with our community of super-women!

Acknowledgments

Granny,

I wish you were still here. I know you would not accept all that I am and have become, but that doesn't change the fact that I wish you could spend more time with your great-grandchildren. They deserve the same kind of joy-filled childhood that I had at your house.

I don't know what happens beyond the grave, but I hope what I told Lennon, about you being with Poppy in Heaven, is right. Say hello to him from us. I don't know if you're looking down on me, or if you get to know what's happening to the ones you left behind, but know that I understand myself better now. I understand *you* better now.

I hope you can see joy radiating from my life. I hope you can see me laugh the way you used to do with my children, and the way you used to do with me. Maybe you're looking down watching me burn the holiday dressing and pointing a crooked finger at me for old times' sake, I don't know.

I hope you're watching my attempts at making chicken and dumplings just like you used to make, with your secret ingredient. I hope you see everything, and I hope even if you don't understand my choices, you accept me and love me. I can't wait to see you again someday.

-Your Sugar Foot

Mom,

Remember the day I came by your house during my lunch break to drop off some groceries? I ran in quickly. Kelsey waited in the car. You sat on a stool in the kitchen, and I stood by the table on the other side of the room. We hadn't spoken of my divorce even though I was nearly nine months into it by then.

I watched you struggle to breathe. Your oxygen tank cords were just a couple of inches from my feet. You told me you'd just been diagnosed with lung cancer, and you didn't seem surprised. It took me right back to holding my breath in your Oldsmobile. The oxygen was the only thing keeping you upright. I watched your hands shake, much like Granny's used to before she died. You were always so nervous, and I tried not to do or say anything to make it worse. But on that day, you gave me an opportunity to tell my side of the story, so I took it.

In that handful of short minutes, I told you I hadn't been happy in my marriage. That I'd just been going through the motions. That I needed sleeping medicine to rest. That in such a big, beautiful home, I still felt alone. I told you more, and more, and more, and before I knew it, I felt better. I could see in your eyes that you understood me. With every head nod, with every validating story, I knew you got it.

"I know how you feel," you said. "For years, I used my bedroom as my place to hide. It's where I went to pretend the world didn't exist. I felt bad because you deserved better, but it was the best I could do."

You started to cry.

"You're better off being alone than being with someone who makes you *feel* alone."

In all the years I tried to connect with you and couldn't, there in that moment, over a cancer diagnosis, a divorce, and an all-around shitty situation, you finally saw me. I'd go through a hundred divorces just to have that moment with you.

I needed it.

That little girl needed it.

My past self needed it.

My current self needs it.

My future needs it.

Finally.

-Your Daughter

Kelsey,

I couldn't haven't written this book without you, but you already know that. I wouldn't be who I am today without you, but you already know that, too. Most importantly, I love you, but you already know that, because you know *me*.

-Your *You*

CLINICAL ACKNOWLEDGMENTS

Dr. Tara Vossenkemper, The Counseling Hub, www.thecounselinghub.com

Rachel Harrison, Trauma Specialists of Maryland, www.traumaspecialistsofMD.com

Katy Kandaris-Weiner, Inner Balance Counseling, www.innerbalanceAZ.com

Jenn Bovee, The Mental Wellness Center, www.thementalwellnesscenter.com

Jessica Schroeder, JS Therapy Group, https://jstherapygroup.com

About the Author

Kasey Compton is a spirited entrepreneur who has embraced all the roadblocks of being a business owner, partner, mother, and friend. She loves using her experiences in life to help others tap into who they truly are.

Kasey welcomes opportunities that allow her to reach others and broaden her impact, such as speaking and presenting from the stage, behind the mic as a podcast guest, and through the stories in her books. She is passionate about connecting and engaging with others, as she feels her purpose in life is to help people find their ability to love themselves in a way that brings true joy and fulfillment.

Kasey designed her mental health practice, Mindsight Behavioral Group, to be highly recognizable, community focused, and profitable, helping underserved populations and focusing on the inner workings of trauma in people's lives.

As a consultant, Kasey uses her analytical and creative skills to help people navigate their entrepreneurial journey. Her specialties include cutting through the clutter to pinpoint the right problem, increasing efficiency, and tapping into a person's highest potential.

She lives in her hometown of Somerset, Kentucky, with Kelsey and their rowdy family of seven. They love spending time together outdoors, taking walks, enjoying Lake Cumberland, or playing with their geriatric German shepherd.

Find her online:
Facebook: @hikaseycompton
Instagram: @hikaseycompton
www.kaseycompton.com/backporchbestie

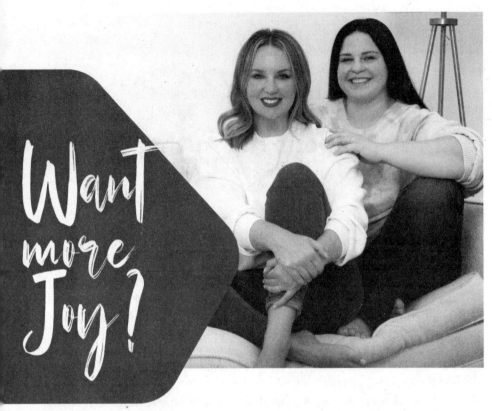

Want more Joy?

The Seeker's Journey

If you're ready to go deeper in the search for joy and inner peace, the Seeker's Journey Online Course is for you. Learn how to communicate with your inner child, understand how your past shapes how you perceive the present, and learn what brings you joy so you can replicate that feeling for the rest of your life.

The Podcast

The Back Porch Bestie Podcast is full of southern wit and wisdom as Kasey and her bestie, Kelsey, discuss life, relationships, and what it means to be a woman, a parent, and a person in the world today. Subscribe to their podcast to never miss a drop of information that can point you toward fulfillment and joy.

 WWW.KASEYCOMPTON.COM

 SEEKER@KASEYCOMPTON.COM

 KASEYCOMPTON.COM/BACKPORCHBESTIE

Kasey Keynotes

Kasey Compton is on a mission to help business owners find their entrepreneurial confidence. Her superpowers include cutting through the clutter to identify strategic starting points, increasing efficiency through systems, and communicating it all in engaging, interactive presentations with tons of heart and Southern charm.

When you hire Kasey to keynote your event, you get:

Actionable Takeaways
Homespun Wisdom
Unforgettable Stories
Relatable Content
Audience Engagement

KASEYCOMPTON.COM/SPEAKING

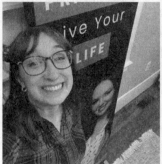
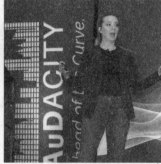
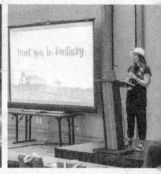